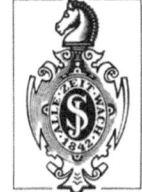

The Dynamic Compression Plate DCP

By M. Allgöwer · P. Matter
S. M. Perren · T. Rüedi

With 26 Figures

Springer-Verlag

New York · Heidelberg · Berlin 1973

Professor Dr. M. Allgöwer,
Vorsteher des Departments für Chirurgie der Universität Basel,
Kantonsspital, CH-4004 Basel

Dr. P. Matter, Krankenhaus, CH-7270 Davos

Priv.-Doz. Dr. S. M. Perren,
Laboratorium für Experimentelle Chirurgie,
Schweizerisches Forschungsinstitut, CH-7270 Davos

Dr. T. Rüedi, Chirurgische Universitätsklinik, CH-4000 Basel

ISBN-13: 978-3-540-06466-4   e-ISBN-13: 978-3-642-65721-4
DOI: 10.1007/978-3-642-65721-4

Typesetting, printing and binding: Universitätsdruckerei H. Stürtz, AG. Würzburg

Contents

General Aspects of the Dynamic Compression Plate (DCP)

The Dynamic Compression Plate (DCP) is an implant for internal fixation of fractures, osteotomies and non-unions. The overall design of the DCP implants is based on the widely used ASIF[1] compression plate system[2]. It can—and in many cases will—be used in exactly the same way as the original ASIF[1] plate, but it offers additional possibilities. The original ASIF[1] instrumentation remains unchanged with the exception of the drill guide. The new design of the compression plate is based on a screw hole design which permits a sliding and a compressive movement during the operation. The design is aimed at increased versatility and easier use.

The DCP may be used for internal fixation of fractures, osteotomies and non-unions in cortical or cancellous bone:

1. as a conventional internal fixation plate (neutralization plate)
2. as a compression plate used together with the removable tension device
3. as a self-compressing plate.

It is important to realize that applications 1 and 2 are identical to those for the ASIF plates ("Müller plates").
Unpredictable load changes on removal of the tension device or upon insertion of screws are prevented by the special screw hole design to be discussed later.
Use as a self-compressing plate should be reserved for cases where exposure is limited, e.g. pelvis, proximal radius.
The need for careful consideration of the indication and exact planning of the operation is unchanged. Internal fixation must always be performed by an experienced surgeon; technical skill and atraumatic treatment of bone, soft tissue, and skin are essential.

Good teamwork and exceptional sterility are further prerequisites. Functional aftercare is an integral part of the treatment of fractures by rigid internal fixation [1].

General Notes on Internal Fixation
The Aim of Internal Fixation

A fracture is a traumatic disruption of the continuity of a bone. Motion at the site of the fracture produces soft tissue irritation and pain. Bony union of the fragments is generally dependent upon immobilization of the fracture site. In "spontaneous healing" this immobilization is achieved by callus formation [2–4], i.e. without rigid fixation

---

1 ASIF = Association for the study of internal fixation.
2 AO = Arbeitsgemeinschaft für Osteosynthesefragen.

by implants. In internal fixation by means of lag screws and compression plates, immediate and absolute immobilization is achieved by interfragmentary compression. Other devices such as wires, intramedullary nails or externally fixed pins are aimed mainly at reducing mobility and improving the position of the bone fragments. In non-union, mere prevention of interfragmentary motion by an implant is often sufficient to cause prompt bone union.

The aim of internal fixation is to allow early, pain-free movement of the injured limb, thus avoiding the sequelae of a long period of immobilization (fracture disease).

Mechanical Basis of Internal Fixation

Changing loads tend to produce relative movement between the fragments. Any such motion results in undesirable fragment shortening due to resorption of bone [5]. Furthermore, relative motion at the fracture site is accompanied by increased mechanical loading of the implant, due mainly to bending and torque. This is especially true if fragment shortening results in loss of bone contact and support. Static forces applied as interfragmentary compression (by the action of the component which acts perpendicularly to the fracture plane) prevent relative movement between the fracture surfaces. Compressive prestress opposing applied tension, and interfragmentary friction opposing shear, prevent relative motion at the fracture site despite the absence of external splinting of the limb during functional follow-up treatment.

Stresses in the plate during functional follow-up treatment may be greatly reduced if the fractured bone is used as a support. This technique necessitates exact reconstruction of the contour of the bone, i.e. the establishment of absolute anatomical continuity and its maintenance as a single block by means of interfragmentary compression whenever possible. The mechanical properties of bone make it well suited to withstand compressional forces. No harm is done to the bone if the "engineering advantages" of compression are exploited up to 200 kp. Contrary to general opinion, static compression does not lead to bone resorption unless motion between contiguous osseous surfaces is allowed to occur.

Biomechanical Basis of Internal Fixation

Biological reaction of living bone to mechanical stimuli (forces and motion) seems to be important in fracture healing. In internal fixation by means of rigid implants, even a minute amount of surface resorption at fragment ends or the screw sites would abolish the rigidity of fixation. Studies have been carried out using compression plates with strain gages providing rigid fixation [6]. These studies have proved that compression applied to living cortical bone is maintained. They exclude the development of even minute amounts of bone resorption at the fracture surfaces [7]. There is abundant proof that, in living bone, it is possible to make use of the engineering advantages of compression fixation without causing adverse bone reaction.

Extensive use of lag screws and compression plates has shown that stabilization of fractures and osteotomies by compression results in relatively fast and effective bone healing. Bone healing occurs faster, when bone vascularity is either maintained or quickly restored. Vascularity of bone is compromised by trauma and by surgical intervention, while revascularization is enhanced by rigid immobilization of the fragment ends [8, 9].

Biology of Bone Healing under Rigid Immobilization

Experimental evidence and clinical experience show that rigid immobilization results in cortical bone healing without the formation of external callus (primary bone healing) [10–13]. When fragment ends in close contact are rigidly fixed by means of interfragmentary compression, they unite by direct bridging with newly formed osteons (contact healing) [14, 15]. Small gaps between fragment ends held in rigid fixation are filled directly by lamellar bone of which the structure is oriented transversely to the long axis of the bone shaft. Bone of this type later undergoes internal remodeling by newly formed osteons (gap healing) [14, 15]. Gaps should be avoided whenever possible, for both mechanical and biological reasons.

Comments on Radiological Follow-Up of Internally Fixed Fractures

The radiological criterion of good healing is not visible callus but disappearance of the fracture line [16]. Any widening of a fracture line which is accompanied by the formation of cloudy callus, pain, and swelling, is indicative of instability and spells danger. In such a case, the reduction of functional load is followed by transformation of the cloudy "irritation" callus into sharply outlined "fixation" callus and simultaneous regression of the pain and swelling.

Problems Associated with Compression Plates Available Hitherto

Some time ago (e.g. LANE [17]) plates were meant to be merely fixed to the bone fragments in a fracture. DANIS [18] recognized the value of interfragmentary compression using plates applied under tension along the longitudinal axis of the bone. His plate contained a built-in compression device (Fig. 1a). MÜLLER [19] designed the ASIF plate with a removable tension device because there was no advantage in leaving the tension device in place after surgery (Fig. 1b). EGGERS [20] tried to exploit the compression effect produced by functional load by the use of elongated holes.
Eccentric placing of screws with conical shoulders to achieve compression is a widely applied principle of carpentry (Fig. 1c). BAGBY [21] designed a plate based on this principle, which produces compression in the longitudinal axis of the bone when the screws are driven home. His design is based on the geometry of the screw with the conical shoulder gliding down the edge of an oval screw hole. Other designs involving self-compressing screw holes based on a conical screw shoulder are the semitubular ASIF plate (Fig. 1d), the plate designed by TAMAY and HOSHIKO [22], and those of

3

DENHAM [23], LUHR [24], and MITTELMEIER [25]. BERTOLINI's [26] plate design is based on oblique insertion of the screws.

Only in the DCP is a spherical geometry applied [27]. Spherical geometry provides a congruent fit between screw and plate in any position along the screw hole, while permitting a certain degree of tilt between screw and plate. Furthermore, the DCP permits a self-compressing action between congruently fitting screw and plate, resulting in compression of the fracture.

Fig. 1   Compression plates available hitherto

    a   The DANIS plate contains a built-in compression device which is not removed during surgery

    b   ASIF compression plate with removable tension device ("MÜLLER plate")

    c   Eccentrically placed screw with conical shoulder to achieve compression is a widely applied principle of carpentry

    d   Semitubular ASIF plate based on conical geometry of the screw shoulder and an oval screw hole

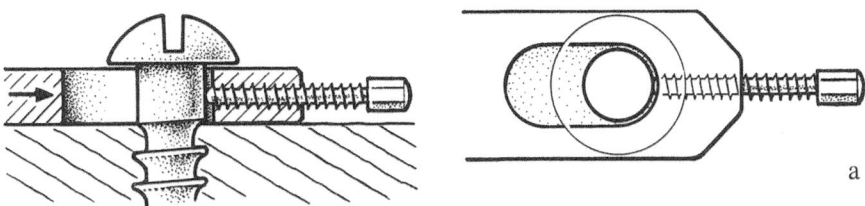

a

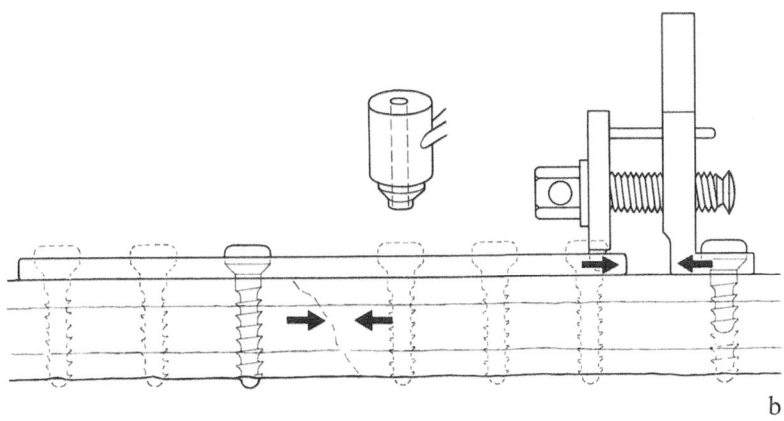

b

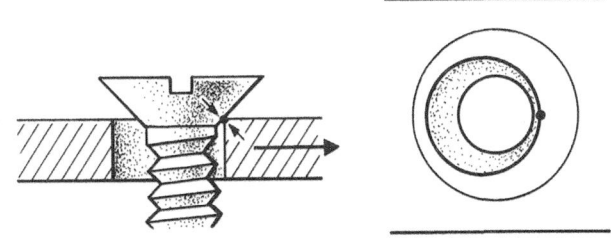

c

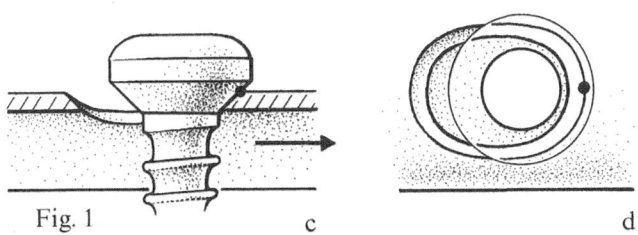

Fig. 1

d

1. Circularly Fitting Screw Holes

a) Unpredictable Load Changes

In a rigid compression plate with a precise circular fit between screw and plate, any additional screw placed after the initial compression will result in unpredictable changes of the compression force. This is due to unavoidable slight eccentricities in the position of the screw. Such changes have been shown to occur even in the hands of a group of 36 skilled surgeons using a precision drill guide (Fig. 2) [28]. Of the 36 surgeons, 17 were found to have achieved zero compression (or distraction) after the application of a four hole plate to intact bone.

b) Lack of Versatility

A close conical fit between screw and plate means the screw always has to be inserted perpendicular to the plate. In some instances, however, it is impossible or disadvantageous to maintain a perpendicular relationship between the screw and the plate. It is always preferable to keep the tip of the screw away from a fracture line. Furthermore, oblique positioning of a screw may be used to increase the force vector perpendicular to the oblique fracture line. Both problems can only be resolved by a spherical fit between plate and screw, which permits a certain degree of tilt between screw and plate in any direction (see also Fig. 14). An incongruent fit between screw shoulder and plate hole results in reduced rigidity of fixation and indroduces unwanted lateral forces between screw and plate.

c) Friction between Screw Head and Screw Hole after Plate Bending

If a plate is contoured to fit a curved bone surface, circularly fitting screw holes on the concave side of the bend will no longer match the screw in diameter. This may produce very high friction which will resist rotation (Fig. 3) [29] and may even prevent the screw from entering the screw hole.

Fig. 2   Compression measurements: Removable tension device, circular snugly fitting screw hole

   a A group of 36 skilled surgeons used a removable tension device to apply compression to an intact femur by means of a modified ASIF compression plate with conical geometry and circularly fitting screw holes. The initial compression and subsequent changes after insertion of all the screws and removal of the tension device were measured

   b Results of experiments outlined in Fig. a. The average initial compression is around 80 kp and shows a wide spread of values. Introduction of the first screw reduced the compression to about 60 kp and resulted in a wider spread of values. In 8 cases "negative compression" (= distraction) was found. At the end of the experiment the average compression value was only 14 kp. In 17 cases no compression was retained. The reason for these changes is slight unavoidable eccentricity in placement of the screw holes, which results in large changes in compression in a comparatively rigid system

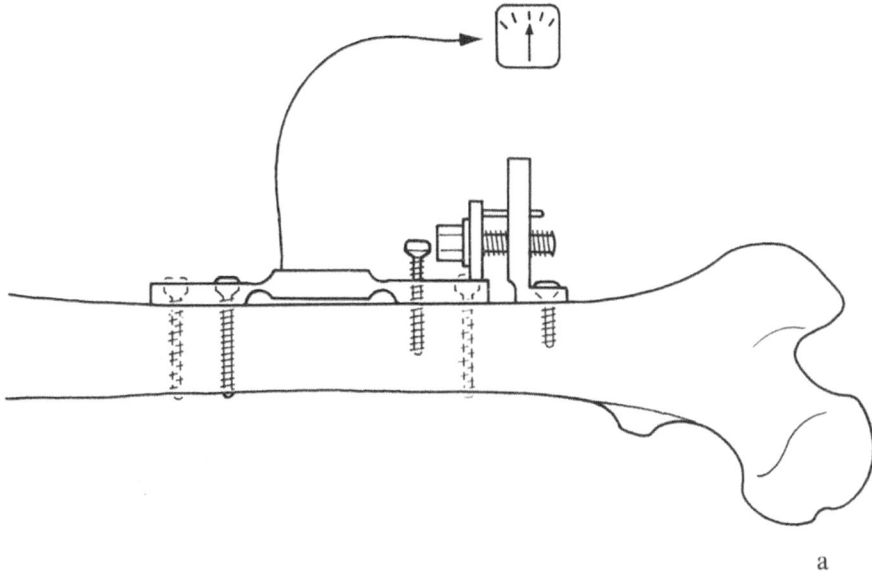

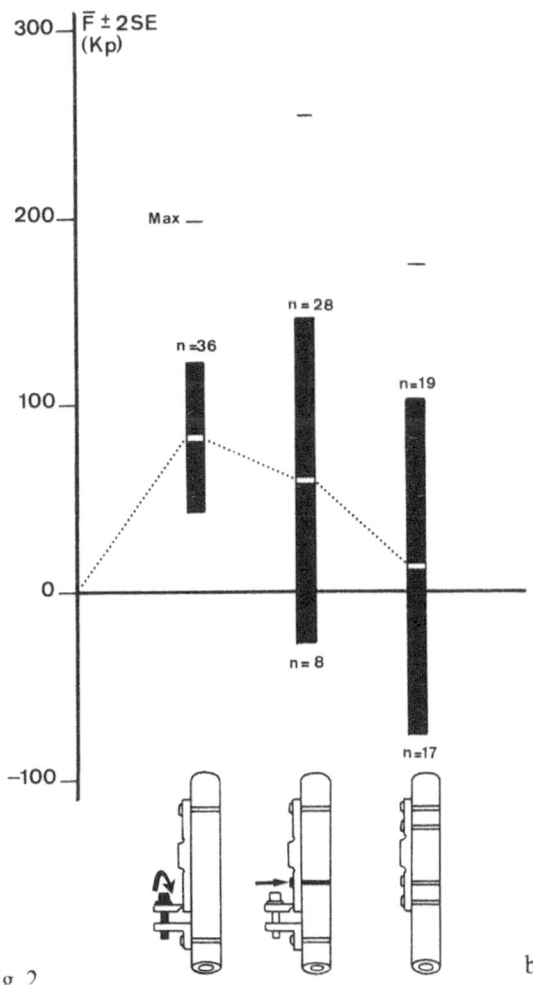

Fig. 2

2. Built-In Tension Devices

a) Metallurgical Hazards

Any built-in tension device increases the number of crevices between opposed metal surfaces. Such crevices are undesirable because they favour corrosion.

b) Lack of Versatility

Optimal treatment of some fracture situations is precluded if it is possible to apply tension at only one screw site.

3. Removable Tension Devices

a) Advantages

The removable tension device offers considerable advantages. It avoids the metallurgic hazards of a built-in tension device and gives a good "feel" for the tension applied. Therefore, we recommend continued use of this device wherever possible.

b) Drawbacks

There are, however, certain drawbacks to the removable tension device:

Extensive Surgical Exposure

Removable tension devices generally require more extensive surgical exposure which may be a problem for example in forearm fractures. Here one would like to use the longest plate possible for a given exposure.

Problems Associated with Compression Applied at the End of the Plate

Slipping of Oblique Fractures. If the angle between the fracture plane and the plate is obtuse towards the tension device, compression applied at the end hole will cause slipping (Fig. 15a).

Kinking or Buckling. A further disadvantage of any end-hole compression is kinking (Fig. 4). It must be counteracted during surgery by clamps, wires etc., a procedure which is likely to increase tissue trauma.

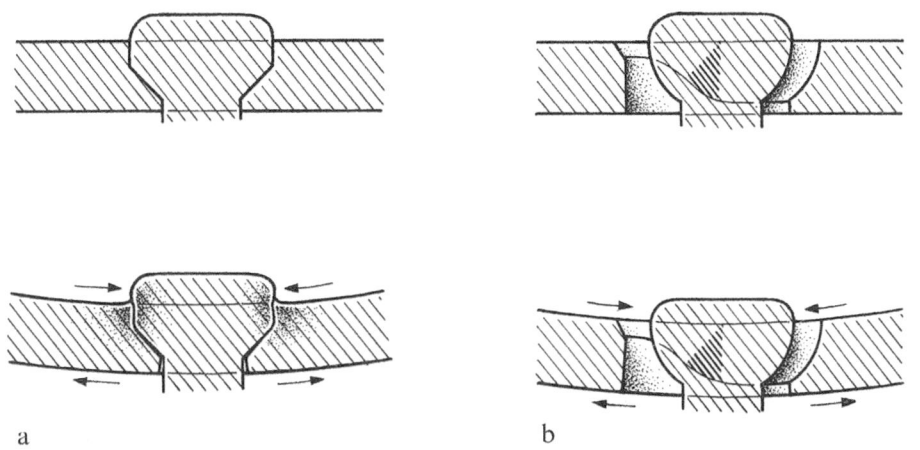

Fig. 3   Effect of contouring a plate with tightly fitting conical screw holes and with the DCP on the screw head

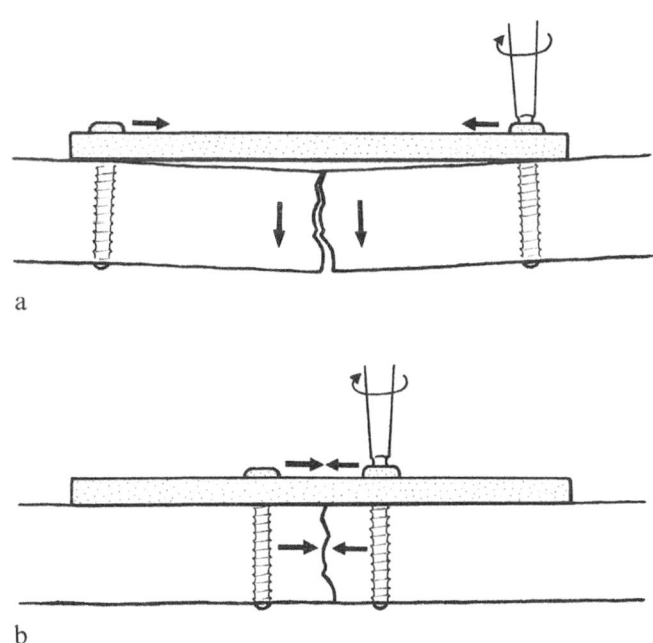

Fig. 4   Buckling associated with tension applied at the plate end

a   Buckling or kinking: When compression is applied from the plate end, whether with a removable tension device or with a self-compressing screw hole, the fracture site tends to give way sideways

b   Compression applied from near the fracture site does not produce this effect

The Concept of Dynamic Compression Plates (ASIF-DCP)

The DCP has been designed to avoid the drawbacks mentioned above. It can be used in a similar way to the other plates, but at the same time it offers a variety of additional possibilities.

The DCP corresponds to the widely tested ASIF plate in overall design and mechanical strength. Only one type of instrument is changed and this is the drill guide, all other instruments remaining identical. The DCP is available as a narrow or a broad straight plate (Fig. 5a and b). The length of the plate depends solely on the number of screw holes. The distances between the screw holes are the same on all DCP's so that plates of different lengths are interchangeable. The distance between the screw holes also permits a change from a conventional ASIF plate to a DCP if necessary.

Tests have shown that the DCP produces the same degree of rigidity of fixation as do optimally applied conventional ASIF plates. In animal experimentation, compression applied to living cortical bone by means of the DCP has been shown to last for weeks and months, like that obtained with the optimally placed conventional ASIF plate [27]. The geometry of the screw holes and screws of the DCP is designed to achieve a congruent fit even when the screw is tilted. Furthermore, the horizontal extension of the screw hole prevents unwanted changes in compression when the screw is in place. Compression of the fracture is produced by driving a screw home after using the special drill guide.

All screw holes are so constructed that any obstruction which would prevent closure of the fracture line is avoided and all screw holes permit a self-compressing action. The space for the shaft of the screw is enlarged in the end holes so that these holes can be used for cancellous bone screws. Shorter plates are provided with one and larger plates with two end holes.

The plate is available in the conventional ASIF steel and in titanium oxygen alloy. With titanium, a more flexible implant material, a comparable degree of mechanical strength may be achieved. Titanium will afford the bone less protection from desirable functional stresses than the hitherto available steel or chromium cobalt alloys. (Whether this helps by giving more physiological signals to the bone, thus preventing "stress-protection osteoporosis" is still open to debate.)

10

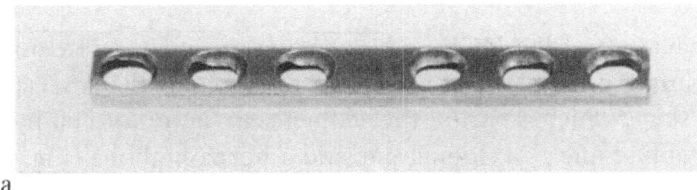

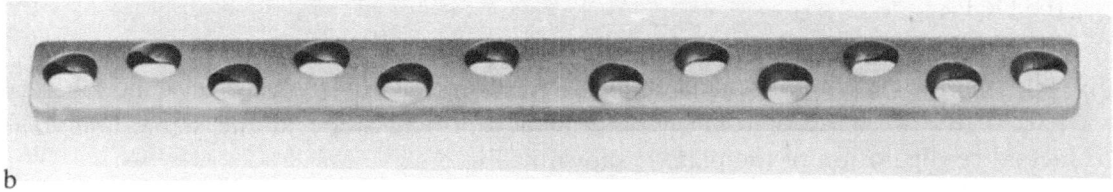

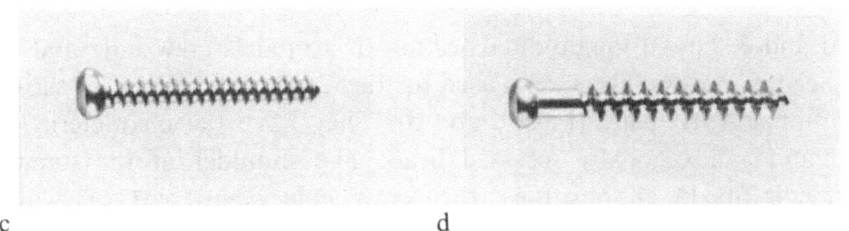

Fig. 5 DCP implants made of steel or titanium-oxygen alloy

a, b Large and small dynamic compression plate, both of which are available in different lengths

c, d Screws for cortical and cancellous bone. These screws are identical to the ASIF/AO screws available hitherto

The Construction of the Dynamic Compression Plate
Screw Hole and Spherical Gliding Principle

The characteristic feature of the DCP is the new design of its screw hole. It is based on the spherical gliding principle. The original screw hole of the ASIF plate (Fig. 1 b) was modified to a shape which is part of the geometrical figure formed by two cylinders intersecting at an obtuse angle: a sloping one and a horizontal one (Fig. 6 a–c).

The principle is best understood by visualizing a ball rolling down an inclined cylinder which meets a horizontal cylinder at the bottom (Fig. 6 a).

Fig. 6 b outlines the part of the two cylinders which forms the actual screw hole in the DCP.

Fig. 6 c demonstrates the initial position of the screw when the DCP is used as a self-compressing plate. Insertion of the screw will displace the plate, because the spherical part of the screw head will meet the hemicylindrical slope of the screw hole. The actual configuration of the plate is shown in Fig. 5.

Design of the Screw Head

Fig. 6 d and e show a longitudinal section of a model screw hole and corresponding "ball-headed" screw. The screws used for the DCP are identical to those used for the conventional ASIF plate (Fig. 5 c and d). They have the characteristic ASIF screw thread and a hexagonally recessed head. The shoulder of the screw is spherical, therefore it fits in all positions, the screw hole being part of cylindrical bodies (Fig. 6 b).

Drill Guide

Three different types of drill guide are used to produce different screw positions in the longitudinal axis of the screw hole. The neutral guide (Fig. 7 a) is the one most often used, and could be called the normal drill guide. It has a central hole which places the screw near the neutral position (the intersection of the two cylinders forming the screw hole). The load guide (Fig. 7 b) places the screw with an eccentricity of 1 mm on the sloping part of the screw hole. The buttress guide (Fig. 7 c) places the screw at the end of the horizontal extension of the screw hole.

Mode of Action

The different positions of the screw relative to the inner contour of the plate hole are seen in Fig. 8.

A screw placed with the neutral drill guide will start in position 8 b and after a minimal compressive movement (0.1 mm) reach position 8 c (the neutral position). From this position the screw can travel towards the fracture but not in the opposite direction.

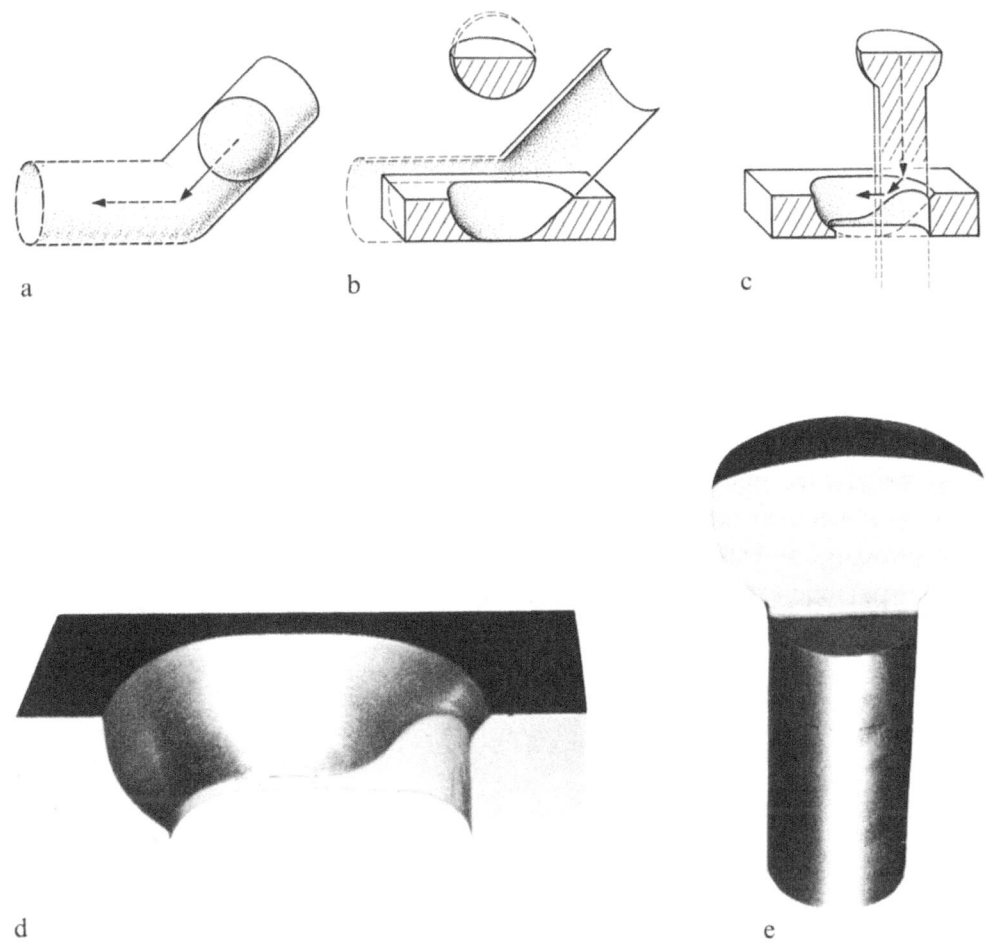

Fig. 6   Spherical-gliding principle

a–c   *Schematic representation*

The new screw hole, which permits compression of the osteotomy (or fracture) when the screw is driven home, offers adequate stability and prevents any locking effect

a   A ball (screw) is guided in a sloping cylinder (screw hole). Any downward movement will result in horizontal displacement. No lateral movement is possible. The position aimed at is the intersection of the two cylinders. This position offers maximal stability without any locking effect. In the horizontal cylinder, displacement towards the osteotomy is possible

b   Projection of the cylinders into the screw hole and the half-shaped screw

c   Actual shape of the hole with the slot necessary for the screw neck and thread

d, e   *Model*

The spherical countersunk screw head is congruent to the hemicylinders constituting the screw hole in any position

d   Longitudinal section through the screw hole of the DCP

e   Longitudinal section through the screw head of the DCP

Closure of the fracture is therefore possible and distraction of the fragment ends is prevented (Fig. 9).

Optimal lateral guidance is ensured throughout this movement. The neutral drill guide is used for all applications of the DCP except when self-compressing action or buttress action are involved. It is therefore the one which is used most often. *We recommend as the normal procedure the one illustrated in Fig. 10.*

A screw placed with the load guide results in compression along the longitudinal axis of the plate when driven home. In Fig. 12 compression is achieved with two screws placed sequentially at one side of the fracture line, the load guide being used for each. The amount of compression achieved is relatively high and uniform. It must be borne in mind that the load on the screw neck is higher in this type of application than when the removable tension device and neutral position of the screw are used.

A screw placed with a buttress guide prevents any further advance of the screw towards the fracture. A screw placed in this way will protect a comminuted area from sintering together. Functional load, together with friction between plate and bone, will impede any movement of the screw in the opposite direction. This guide should be used only exceptionally, and should never be turned around and used for additional compression, as this puts too much stress on the screw.

Fig. 7   Drill guides

a   *Neutral drill guide:* This drill guide is used for application of the DCP in almost all cases except when screws with self-compressing or buttress action are to be used. Screws placed with the aid of this drill guide meet the sloping cylinder near the final screw position. Minimal additional compression results. This drill guide is green, indicating that its use is recommended most of the time

b   *Load guide:* A screw placed with the aid of this drill guide meets the sloping cylinder 1 mm from the final position. If good adaptation has been achieved, 60 kp compression may be obtained when inserting the screw after use of this drill guide. The yellow colour indicates that the load guide should be used with caution

c   *Buttress guide:* A screw placed with the aid of this drill guide meets the screw hole at the end of the horizontal extension. The screw can therefore not travel any further towards the fracture. This drill guide is used in situations where it is necessary for the fracture to be supported by means of the plate. This drill guide is red, indicating that it should be used with extreme caution. We strongly discourage reversal of the drill guide to increase the self-compressing action over a longer distance, because this may put too great a strain on the neck of the screw

---

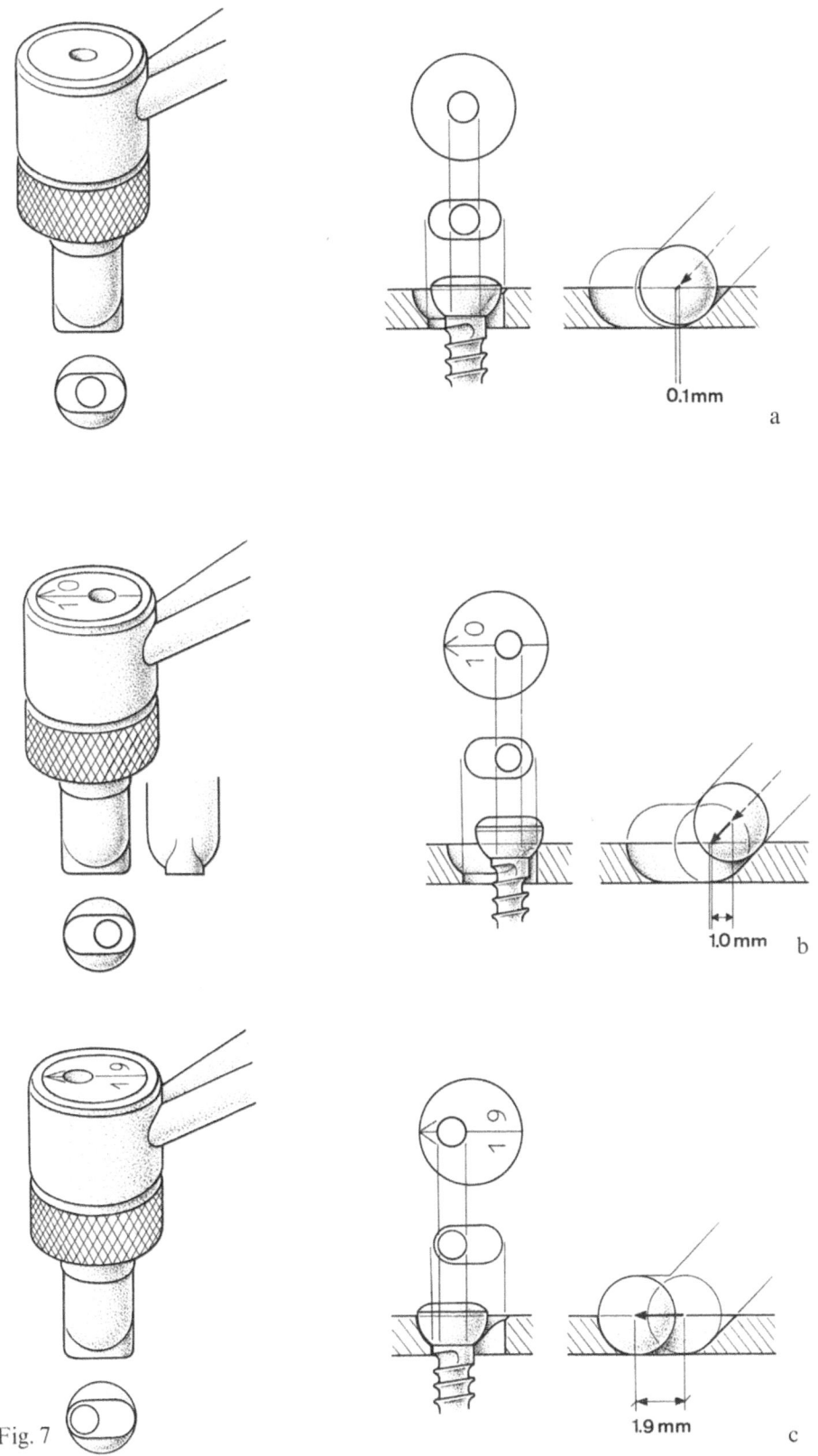

Fig. 7

a

0.1mm

b

1.0 mm

c

1.9 mm

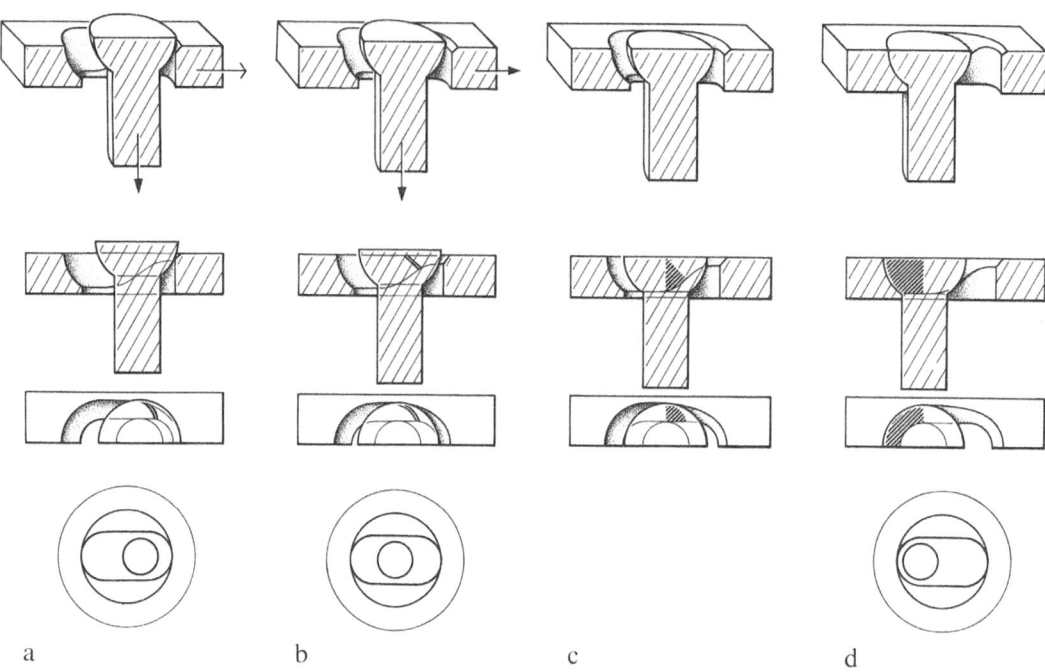

Fig. 8   Relative positions of screw and screw hole. Line and area of contact at different positions seen from the side and from above, and cross-section through the corresponding drill guide

   a   The load guide places the screw 1 mm from the final position on the sloping cylinder. The resulting line of contact is semicircular

   b   The neutral guide places the screw 0.1 mm from the final position on the sloping cylinder; a larger semicircular line of contact results

   c   Final position: This is the final position of the screw when internal fixation is complete. It provides an area of contact between screw head and plate which constitutes part of the surface of a sphere

   d   The buttress guide places the screw at the end of the horizontal extension of the plate hole; the screw cannot travel any further towards the fracture

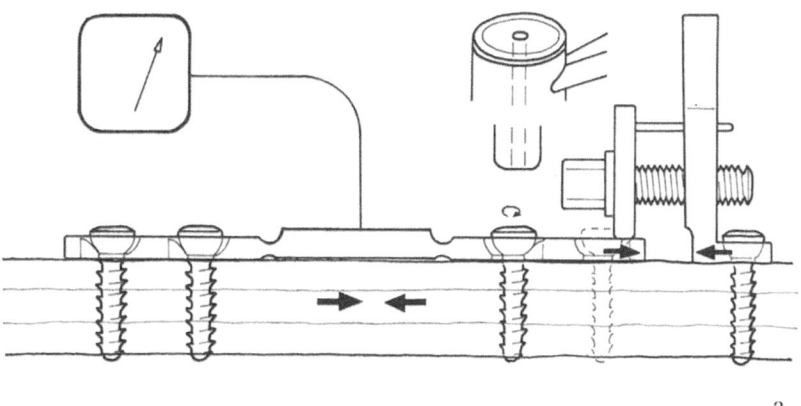

a

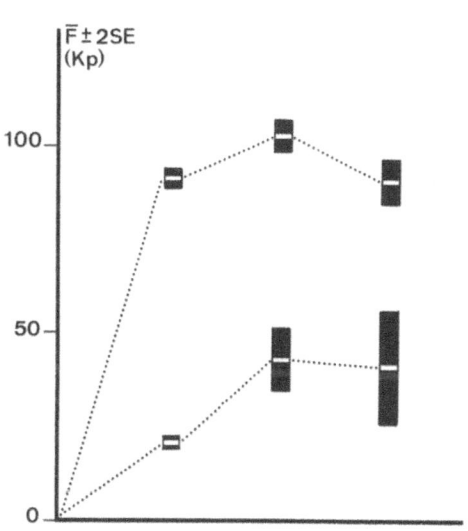

Fig. 9   Compression measurements. DCP with removable tension device

a   Experimental set-up for determination of the amount of compression achieved by use of the DCP with a removable tension device. An investigation was carried out under laboratory conditions, in which 6 consecutive determinations were made at different levels of initial compression. When an instrumented DCP, thc removable tension device, and the neutral drill guide were employed, the compression achieved was monitored during the introduction of the different screws and the removal of the tension device. No loss of compression such as was seen in the investigation illustrated in Fig. 2 occurred in this investigation, because a locking action of the screw is impossible except when the buttress drill guide is used

b   The values for 20 kp and 90 kp were selected from various levels of initial compression. Driving home the screws with a neutral drill guide results in some additional compression which is more marked when the initial compression is low. After removal of the tension device, seating the remaining screws results in only slight reduction in compression, especially at higher compression levels. This compares favorably with the findings illustrated in Fig. 2

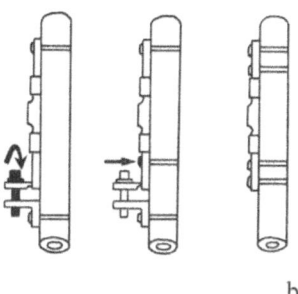

b

17

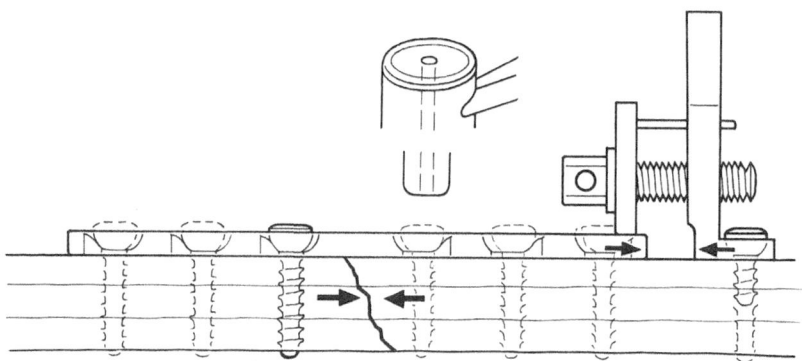

Fig. 10   "Classic application" of the DCP with the removable tension device and the neutral drill guide for all screws. The advantage of this application over circularly fitting screw holes is the maintenance of compression and congruent fit of screws inserted obliquely

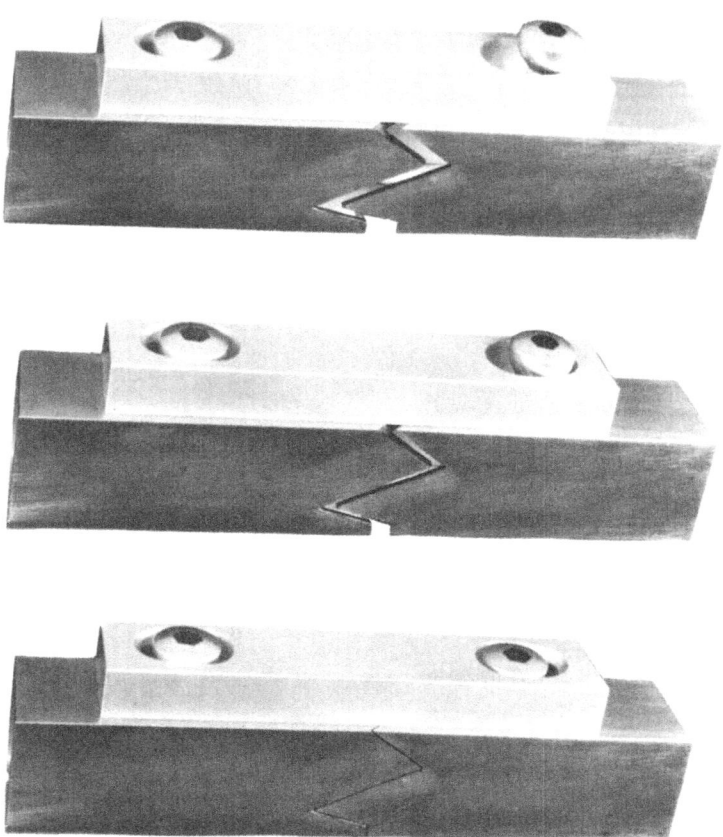

Fig. 11   The model shows the action of the DCP screw hole as a self-compressing screw hole. Driving home the screw results in adaptation and compression of the fracture

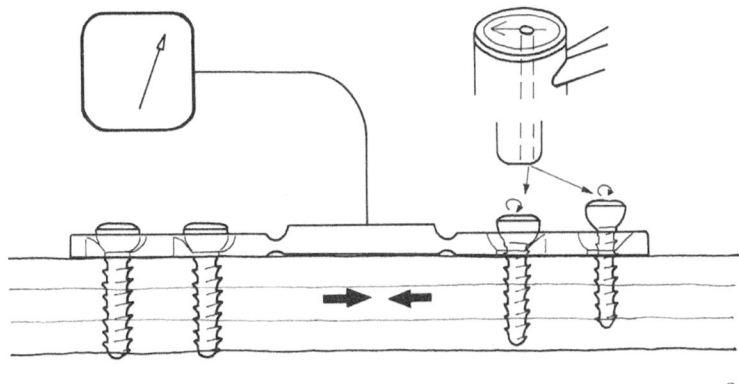

a

Fig. 12 Compression measurements. The DCP as self-compressing plate

a Experimental design used to measure the compression produced by driving home two screws positioned with the aid of the load drill guide

b The initial compression achieved with one screw positioned with the load guide is 60 kp; positioning a second screw with the help of the load drill guide increases compression. Final tightening of the screws results in a slight further increase. It must be borne in mind that the self-compressing action results in a higher bending load on the screw neck than that imposed by the application of a screw in the neutral position or in a conventional plate

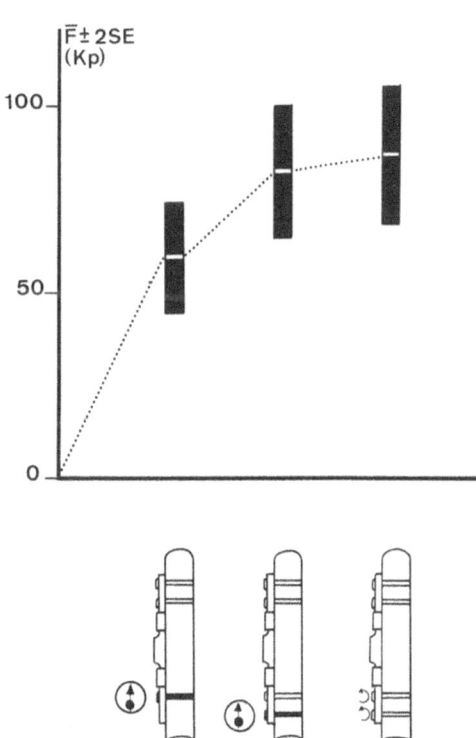

b

Application of the Dynamic Compression Plate

General Considerations

The DCP is applicable in all situations in which a plate is indicated and it is used according to the principles laid down in the ASIF Manual. Whenever possible, it should be placed as a tension band plate, usually on the opposite side to where the strongest group of muscles of the limb is situated.

DCP as a Conventional Internal Fixation Plate

The DCP used with the so-called neutral drill guide (see page 19) does not require any new application technique. After exact reduction of the fracture the fragments are held in place by means of clamps, wires or lag screws. The plate is then contoured to the surface of the bone by bending and twisting. The screw holes are drilled and tapped according to standard ASIF techniques with the aid of the neutral drill guide (Fig. 13). The screws are then inserted and tightened. When a plate of this type is combined with plate-independent lag screws, it protects the lag screw which compresses the fracture line and may be considered as a neutralization plate.

In this application the DCP offers advantages due to the possibility of tilting the screws (Fig. 14), both for the reasons mentioned above and because the screw hole is designed to prevent longitudinal distraction by eccentrically placed screws.

DCP as a Conventional Compression Plate with Removable Tension Device

The DCP is especially recommended for plating of short femoral and tibial fractures and stabilization of cases of non-union, exept for the middle third of the shaft where medullary nailing may be preferable.

Fractures which become stable when compressed in the longitudinal axis of the bone may be treated with the DCP. The fracture is reduced and the plate properly contoured. One screw is placed ~12 mm ($^1/_2''$) from the fracture on one side (the screw may be positioned with the neutral drill guide, thus holding the plate against the bone). The tension device is applied by conventional ASIF techniques. Slight initial tension will align the plate and the tension device. After alignment the screws of the tension device and of the plate are driven home and the bone is compressed by means of the tension applied with the tension device. After insertion of the screws on both sides of the fracture, using the neutral drill guide for each screw, the tension device is removed and the last screw inserted.

The advantages of the DCP in this type of application are that no screw can prevent the closure of the fracture line during the operation and unwanted changes of compression are minimized (Fig. 8). Buckling (Fig. 4) due to "end-hole compression" is prevented by insertion of a gliding screw near the fracture on the side of the tension device (Fig. 15).

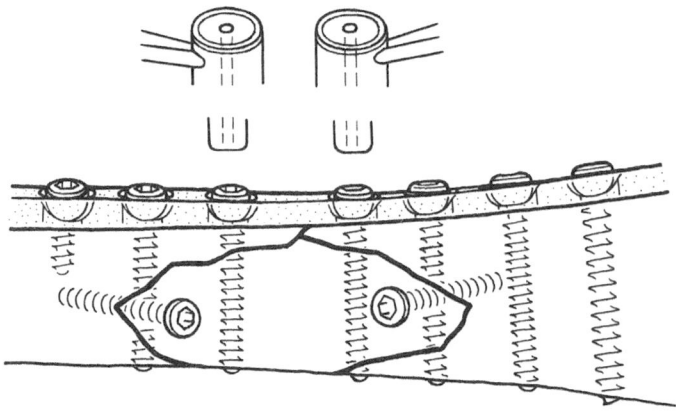

Fig. 13 Application of the DCP as a "conventional" internal fixation plate. The neutral drill guide is used. The advantages of the DCP over other plate designs in this application are the small and uniform preload of all screws and the possibility of introducing screws obliquely

DCP as a Self-Compressing Plate

In certain circumstances, e.g. forearm fractures, the additional exposure necessary for application of the removable tension device may be difficult to obtain. To cope with this situation, the DCP has been provided with self-compressing holes. As noted above, the compression process of the DCP is based on the so-called spherical gliding principle.

The fracture is reduced and the plate is contoured to fit the bone surface (Fig. 16). The plate is then secured to one of the main fragments by means of a first screw near the fracture. The second screw hole is positioned in the opposite fragment using the load guide, also near the fracture. Driving home the second screw will result in compression of the fracture as the fragments are pushed towards each other. Further screws are then positioned with the neutral guide.

In this application, the DCP offers the advantage of maximal exploitation of the available exposure for fixation purposes. Furthermore, compression may be achieved in any screw hole. This feature helps to prevent buckling and enhances the versatility; for example, it is possible to align a comminuted fracture by several gliding screws, adding compression only at the end or sequentially.

DCP as a Buttress Plate

If the screw is placed at the end of the screw hole nearest to the fracture site, the plate will act as a support, e.g. for metaphyseal fractures. The fracture is reduced and all screws are placed in the locking position using the buttress guide (Fig. 17). In this application the DCP permits the same buttress action as the conventional plate but allows additional versatility in placement of the screws (Fig. 14).

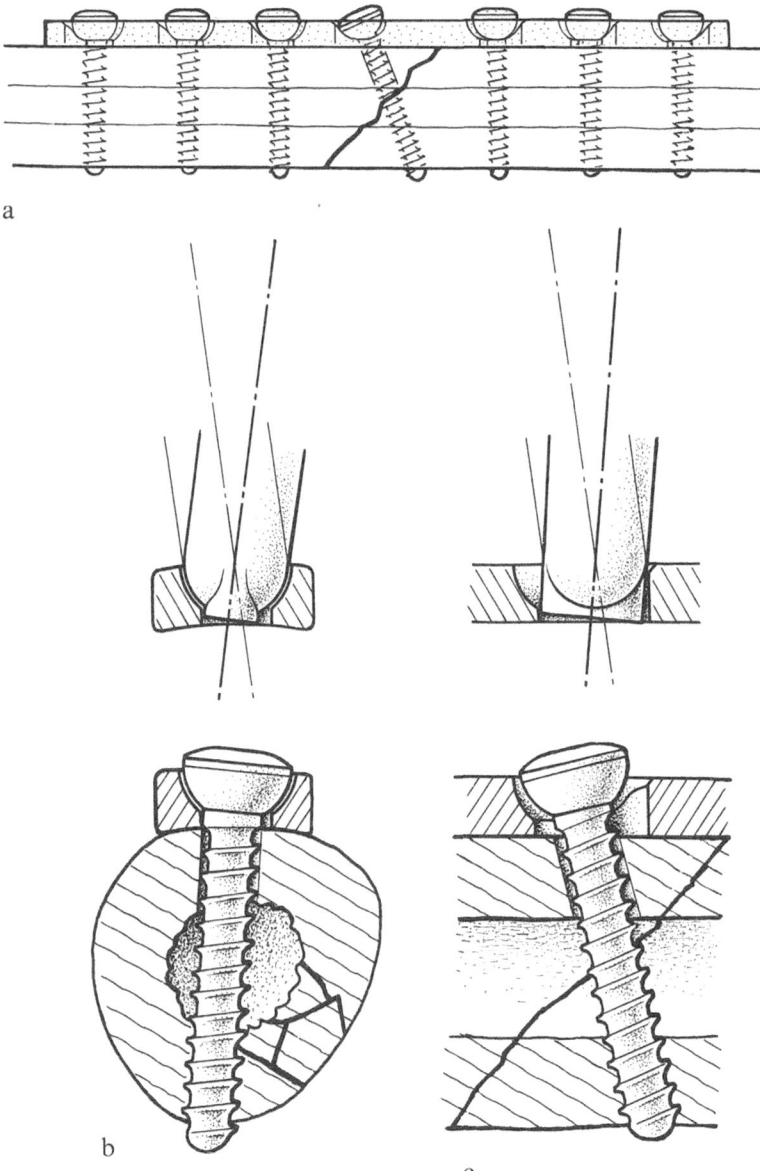

a

b

c

Fig. 14   Advantage of the spherical geometry

a   The design of the screw hole based on the spherical-gliding principle permits tilting of the screws over a wide range along the longitudinal axis of the bone. The spherical-gliding principle maintains a congruent fit between the spherical screw head and the cylindrical screw hole. In this case a screw through the plate is used as a lag screw to achieve interfragmentary compression perpendicular to the fracture line. It is important to realize that interfragmentary compression is a most important means of stabilization in internal fixation

b   Cross-section through the drill guide, which centers the screw head even if the screw is tilted to avoid a comminuted fracture area with the screw tip. Centering the screw head rather than the screw neck prevents unwanted lateral forces between plate and screw

c   Longitudinal section through a drill guide and screw within the plate. A similar application to that in Fig. 14a is shown in the enlargement

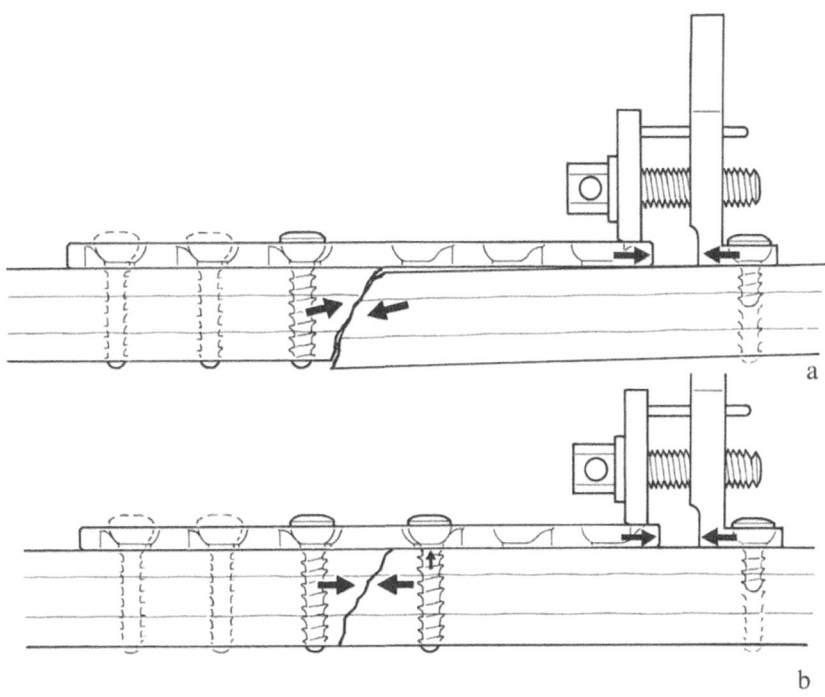

Fig. 15   Prevention of kinking and buckling

    a   In oblique fractures the tension device should be placed as shown in Fig. 1b to prevent a lateral displacement during tightening. In some cases the tension can only be applied from one end of the plate since longitudinal compression may result in a tendency to slip

    b   The DCP makes it possible to introduce a screw near the fracture site, placing it loosely first to prevent buckling while still allowing sliding. The elliptical holes of the DCP permit the first, loosely applied, screw near the fracture site to slide during compression. This screw prevents buckling

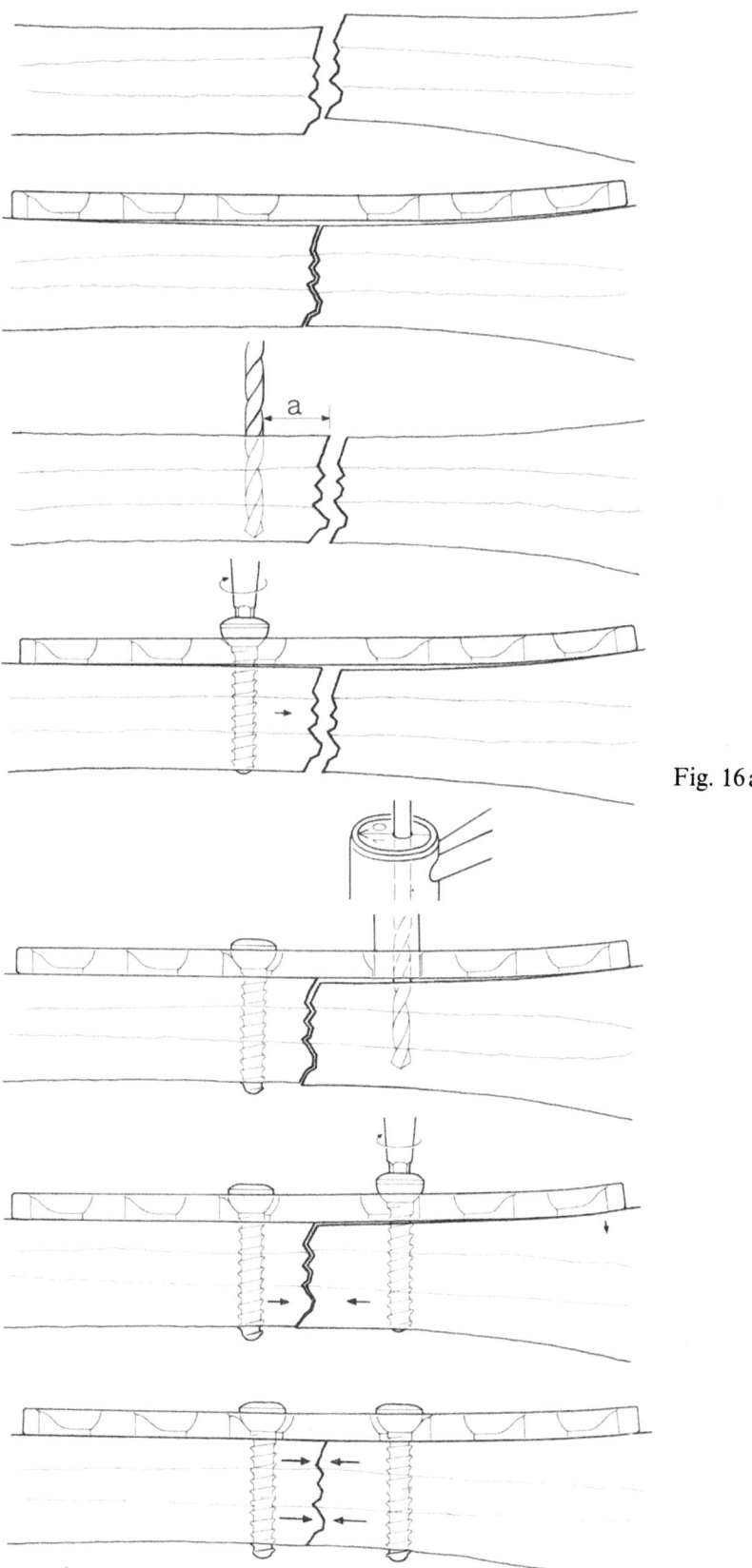

Fig. 16 a

Fig. 16 b

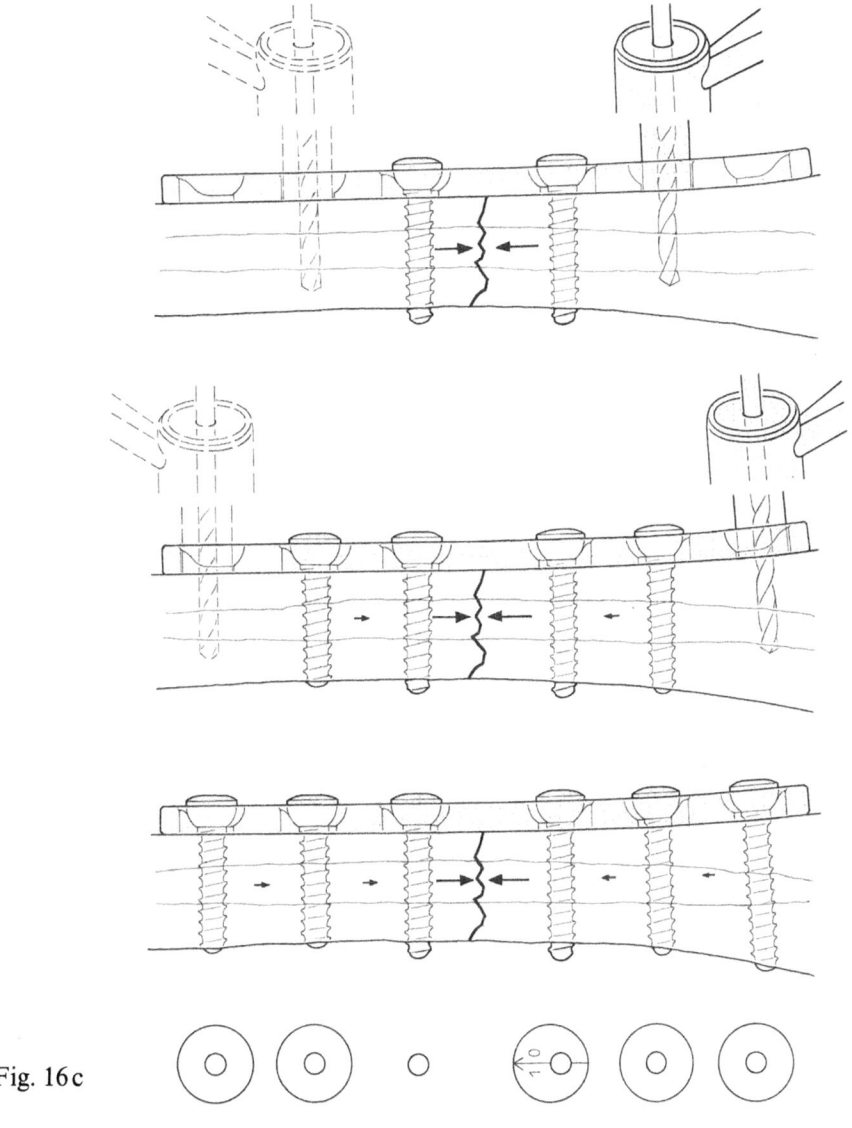

Fig. 16c

Fig. 16   Application of the DCP as a self-compressing plate
a–c
The fracture is reduced and the plate is contoured to fit the bone surface by careful bending and twisting. (If the opposite cortex is not comminuted, the plate is bent so as to cause slight concavity over the fracture site.) The plate is then secured to one of the main fragments by means of a first screw near the fracture. The first drill hole should be placed about 1 cm from the fracture site. The neutral drill guide is used, while the plate is held in place with a forceps or a cerclage wire. The second screw is placed in the opposite fragment but with the aid of the load guide. Driving home the second screw will result in compression of the fracture as the fragments are pushed towards each other. The remaining screws are inserted with the aid of the neutral guide

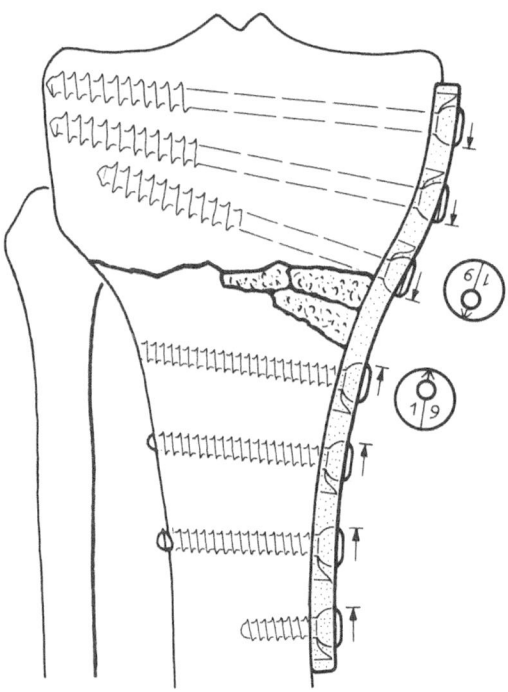

Fig. 17 The use of the DCP as a buttress plate

In cases where the function of the plate is to support, i.e. to prevent sintering together of a comminuted fracture area, the drill holes are placed with the aid of the buttress guide as shown here

Practical Examples

Short Fractures with Direct Contact between the Main Fragments

1. Use of the DCP with the Removalbe Tension Device

Application of the DCP with the removable tension device is recommended whenever adequate exposure is possible and no slipping or buckling is likely to occur. A good practical example is illustrated by the X-ray shown in Fig. 18. The first hole is drilled near the fracture, the plate is contoured to fit the bone and fixed to one fragment with one screw. The tension device is then fixed to the other fragment. After precise alignment of the fracture, the tension device is tightened firmly and the rest of the screws are positioned using the neutral guide. The use of the DCP in combination with the tension device is especially recommended for plating of a femur or tibia.

2. Use of the DCP as a Self-Compressing Plate

This application is recommended when only limited exposure is available (Fig. 16). After preliminary adaptation of the fragments the plate position is selected and the first hole is drilled $^1/_2$ inch from the fracture line. The thread is cut and the first screw is fixed loosely to the plate. The second hole is drilled in the other fragment through the plate hole nearest to the fracture line, using the load guide. Tightening of both screws produces compression at the fracture site. A slight correction of reduction is still possible during compression. Since the compression effect is obtained in the proximity of the fracture, angular displacement of the fragments under compression is avoided. Unsatisfactory reduction of the fragments can be detected by X-rays before addition of the other screws using the neutral drill guide.

Only in exceptional cases is it desirable to increase the compression by inserting further screws with the aid of the load guide. Normally only one screw is inserted by means of the load guide. If additional screw holes are drilled with the aid of this guide the previous screws should be loosened slightly before applying compression with the additional screw.

Torsion or Bending Fractures with Butterfly Fragment

As a first step, screw fixation using lag screws is recommended prior to the application of a neutralization plate. (If a butterfly fragment is present in the cortex opposite to the plate, preliminary fixation with a cerclage wire may be more practical.) In such a fracture, fixation is primarily achieved by lag screws inserted both independently and through the plate. The plate only acts as further protection—a so-called neutralization plate. In a neutralization plate all screws may be inserted in the neutral position with the neutral drill guide. Since "neutral" screw position results in compression

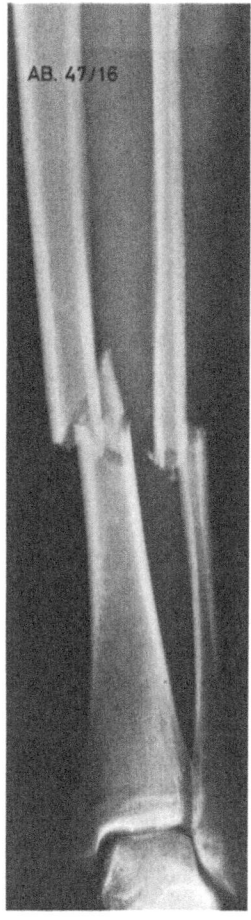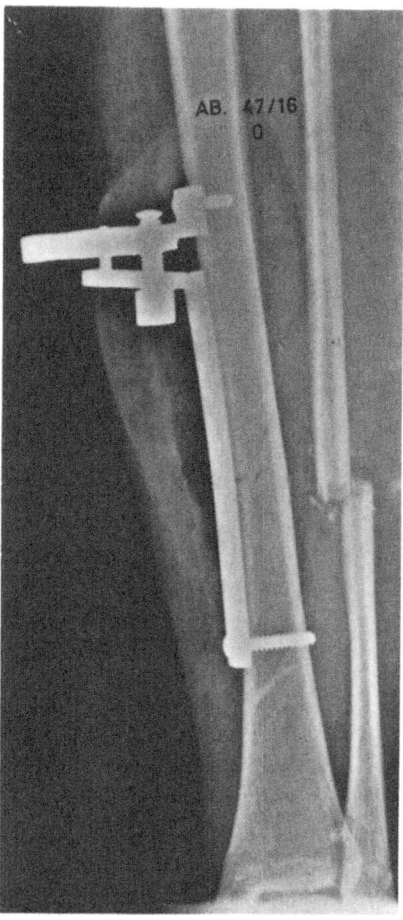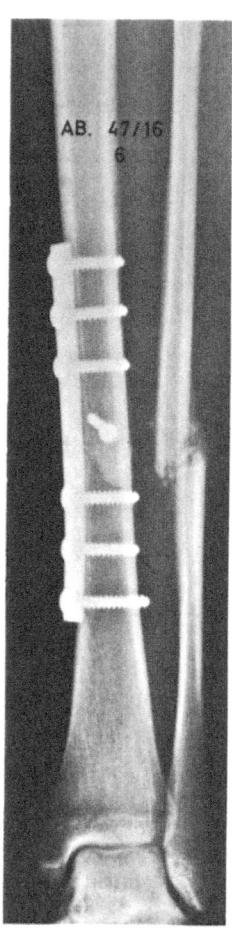

Fig. 18 DCP with the removable tension device

This application corresponds exactly to the one for the hitherto available ASIF plate. The neutral drill guide is used throughout. The advantage is more uniform sustained compression and the possibility of tilting the screws while maintaining spherical contact produced by the 0.1 mm compressive movement, a plate will apply some axial compression to the underlying diaphysis. All screws crossing a fracture line must be applied as lag screws (Fig. 19).

Comminuted Fractures

In these cases the method recommended is preliminary reduction of the comminuted area by means of bone clamps and/or temporary cerclage wires or lag screws, after which the plate will be loosely fixed to the bone (Fig. 20). Since every hole in the plate may be used for compression, it is possible to institute axial compression only when the fragments are fully aligned, thus achieving optimal coaptation of the fragments. Plate screws traversing a fracture line must be applied as lag screws.

Fractures at Two or More Levels

A long plate may be used to span multiple fractures. Any part of the fracture amenable to axial compression may thus be fixed by successive screws, avoiding badly comminuted areas. The DCP is especially well suited to fixation of two-level diaphyseal fractures (Figs. 21 and 22).

Forearm Fractures

Fractures of one or both forearm bones are very suitable for plate fixation in general and with the DCP in particular. This application has already been outlined. Two examples are shown in Figs. 23 and 24.

If a double forearm fracture is to be treated, the simpler fracture is fixed first with two plate-screws. The second fracture is then approached. If reduction of the second fracture is hampered by the fixation of the first, the preliminary fixation of the first can easily be loosened. Complete fixation of each fracture by insertion of the remaining screws is performed only after reduction and preliminary fixation of both fractures.

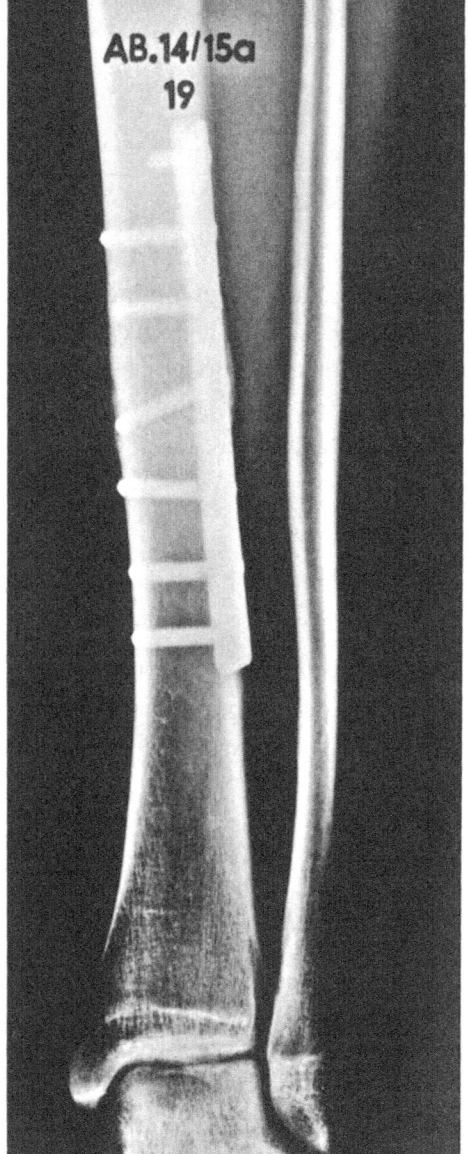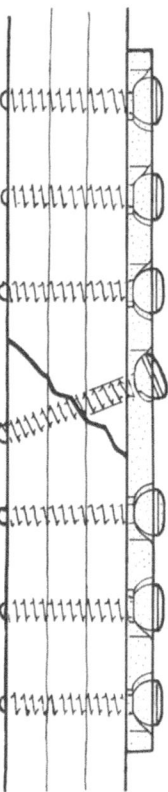

Fig. 19 Application of a lag screw through the DCP in a short oblique fracture of the tibial shaft

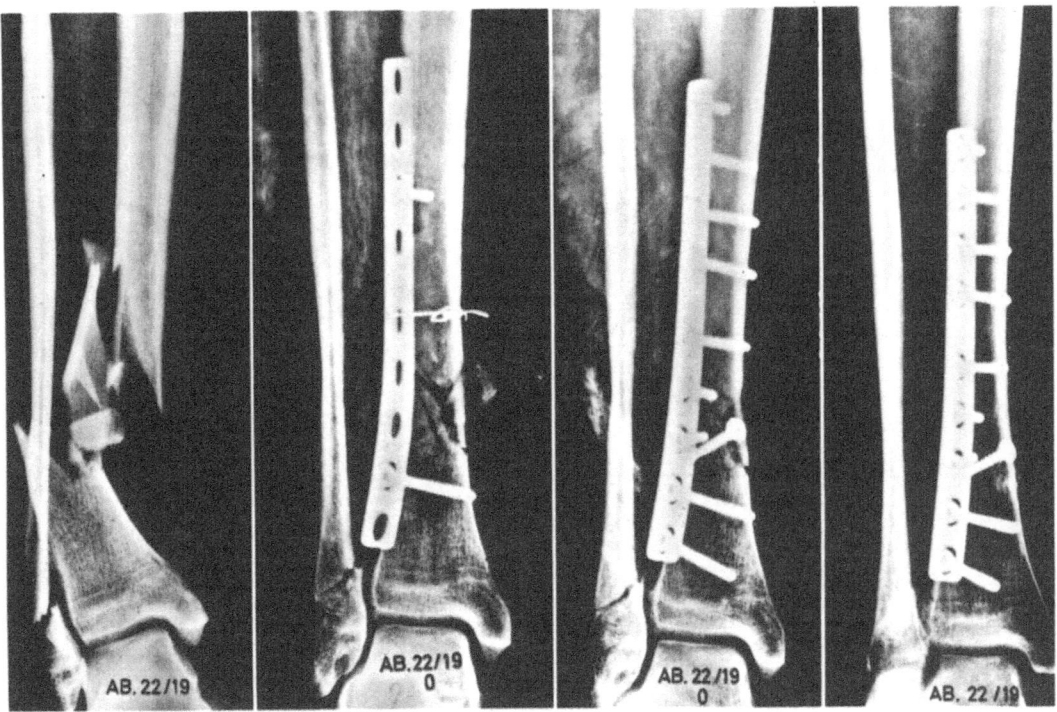

Fig. 20 Comminuted fracture of the lower third of the tibia

Temporary fixation with a cerclage wire, application of the DCP after exact contouring to fit the bone surface. In this exceptional case the plate has been placed laterally instead of medially because of contused skin over the medial surface

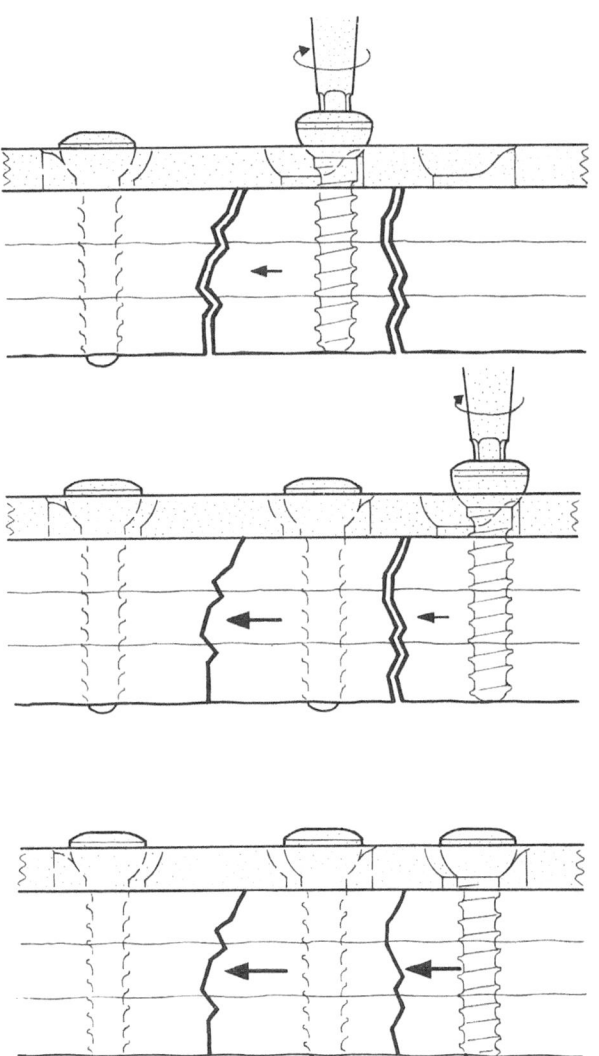

Fig. 21   Fractures at two levels

The DCP is used here as a self-compressing plate permitting the Simultaneous compression of two fractures

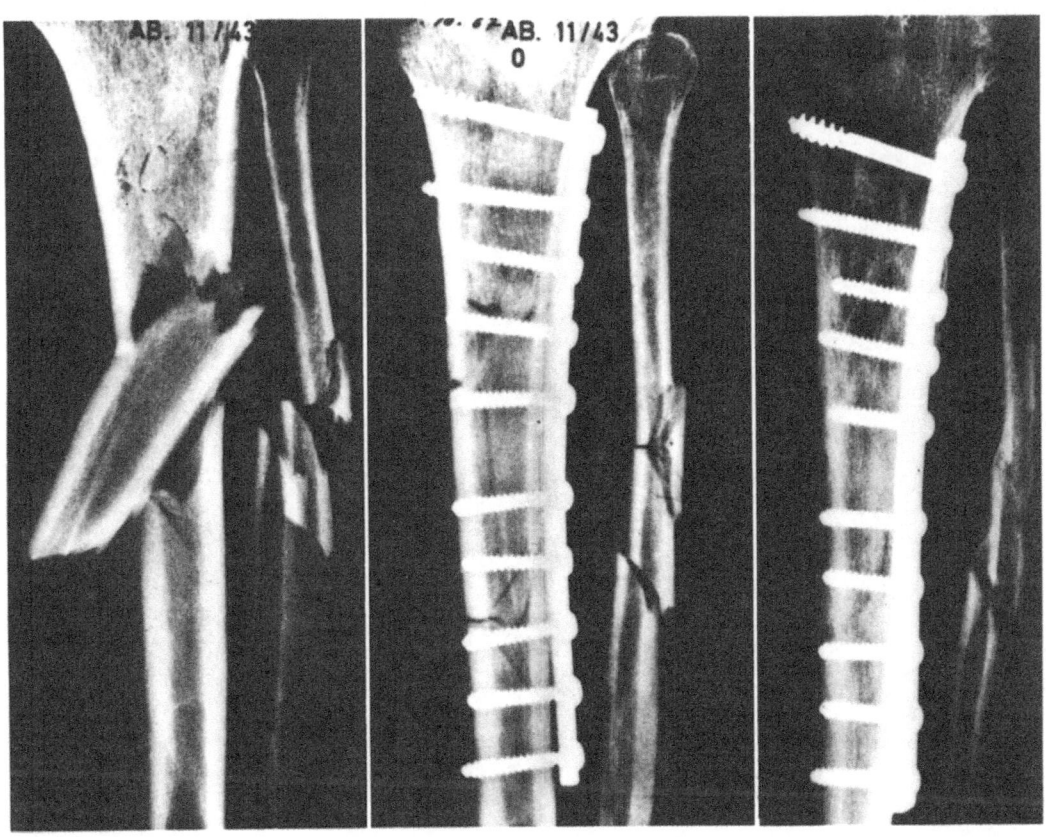

Fig. 22   Clinical application of the DCP in a proximal two-level fracture of the tibia. The proximal end hole is fitted with a cancellous bone screw

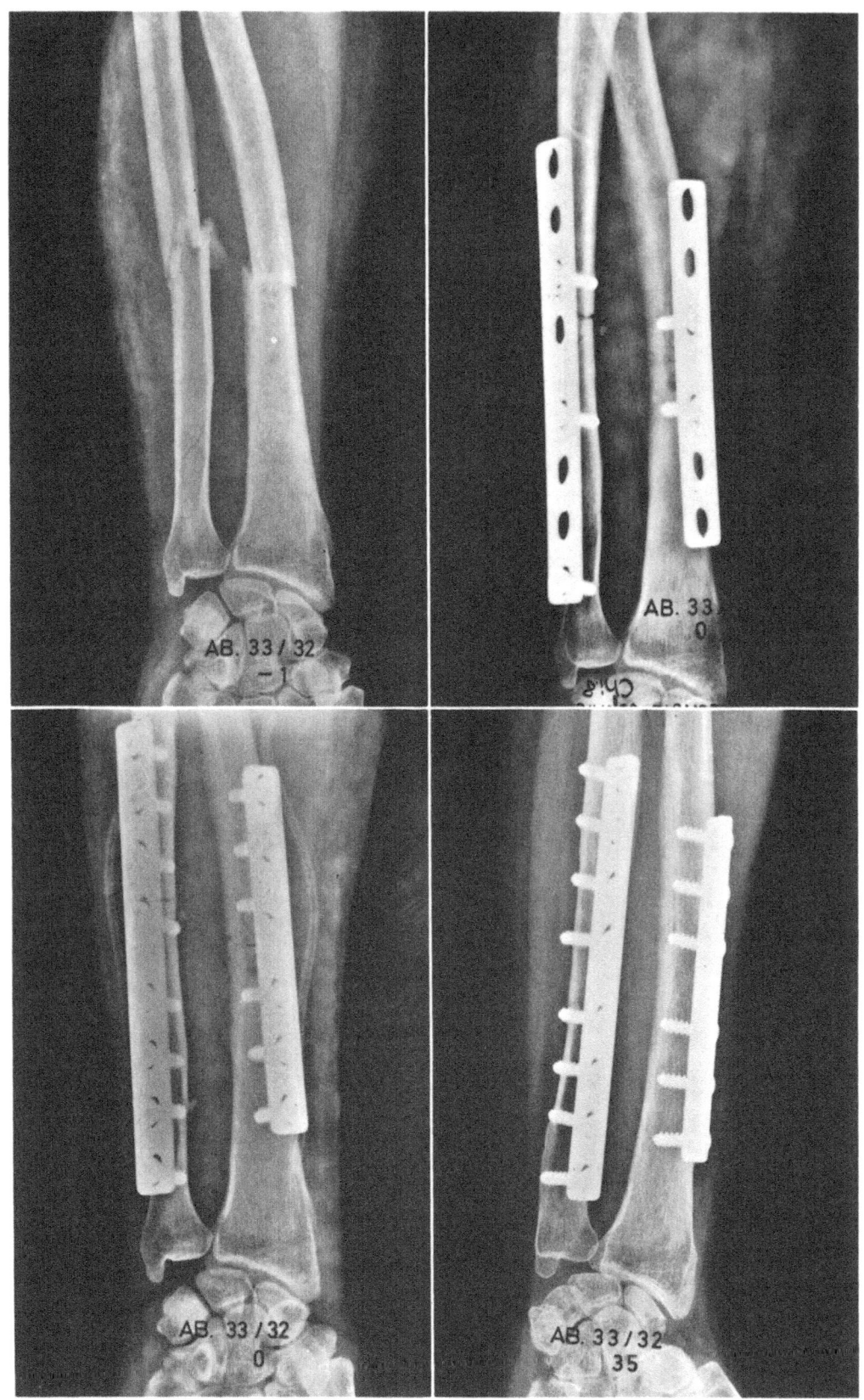

Fig. 23   Legend see opposite page

Fig. 24 Fracture of both forearm bones ▷
treated with a DCP and free lag
screw. Note the plate length.
Forearm fractures should never
be fixed with 4-hole plates

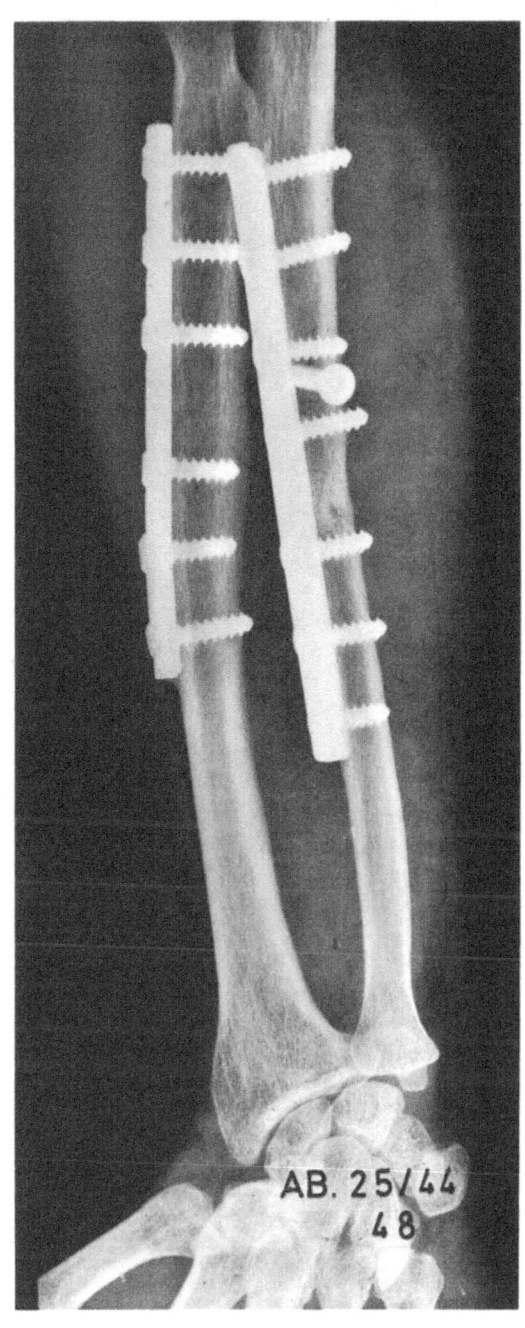

◁

Fig. 23   Treatment of a forearm fracture

The first fracture is secured temporarily with two screws, then the second fracture
is reduced and secured. The temporary fixation of the first fracture with only two
screws permits loosening of the first one during reduction of the second fracture
if necessary. Subsequently, all screws are driven home

Acetabular Fractures of the Pelvis

In acetabular fractures, when exposure is very limited, the possible advantages of the DCP are evident: it facilitates self-compression even of extensively bent plates, and it permits oblique screw positions (Figs. 25 and 26).

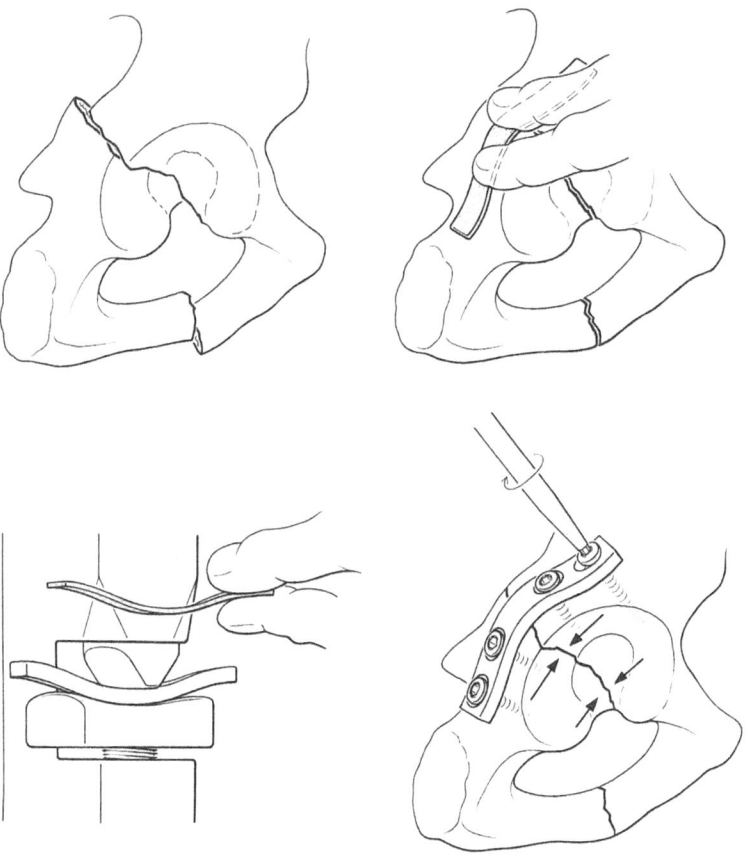

Fig. 25   Diagrams illustrating fixation of an acetabular fracture with a DCP

        The fracture is first reduced, then a small template is contoured to the bone surface by pressure applied with the finger tips. In this application the DCP, used as a self-compressing plate, allows compression where it would be impossible to apply the removable tension device. If the screws must be tilted the spherical screw-hole geometry still permits perfect fit between screw head and plate hole

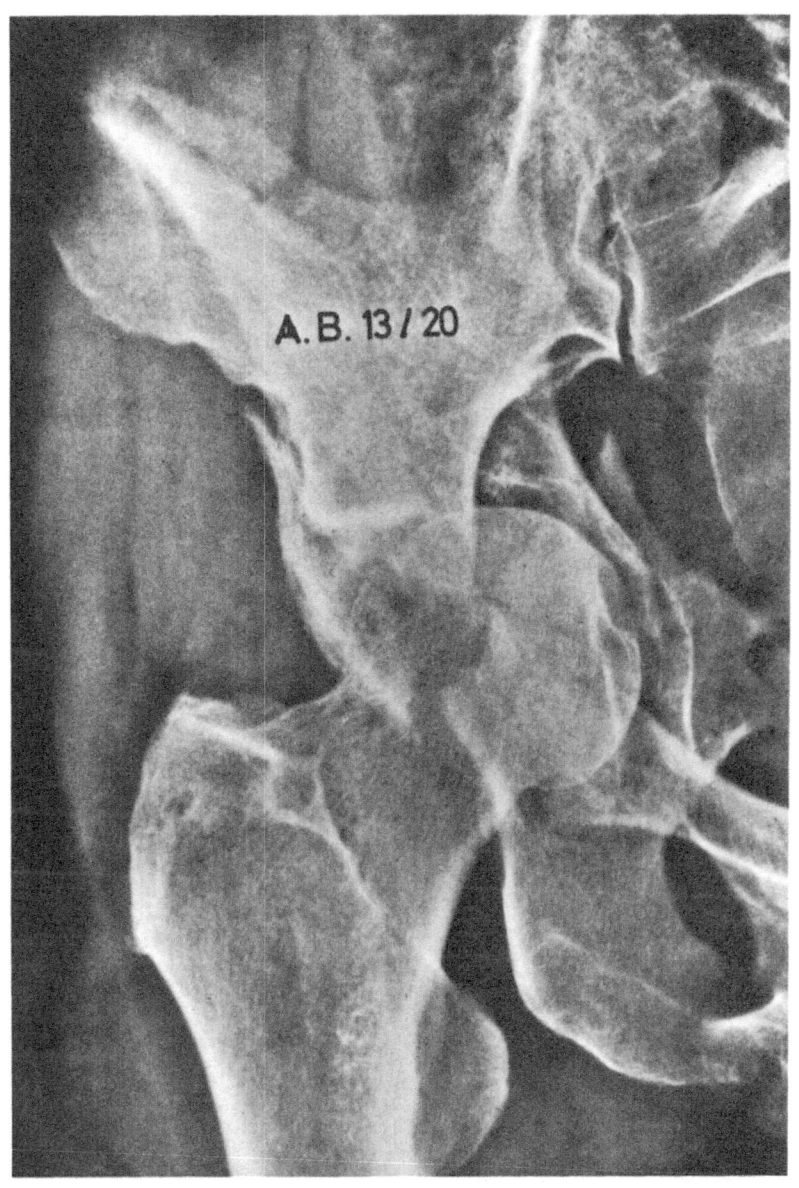

Fig. 26a   Pelvic fracture with central dislocation

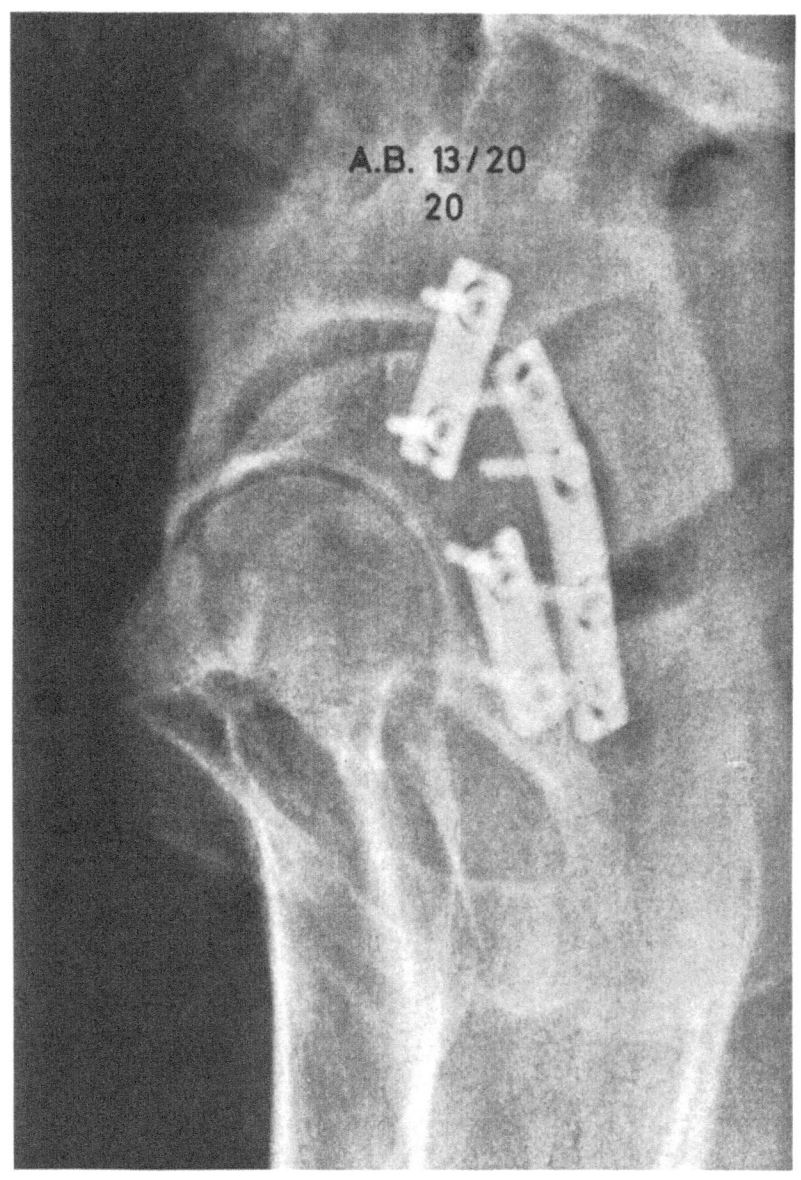

Fig. 26b   Pelvic fracture with central dislocation, fixed with three short DCPs used as self-compressing plates. Perfect realignment of the acetabular region. The illustration shows the fracture 20 weeks after surgery

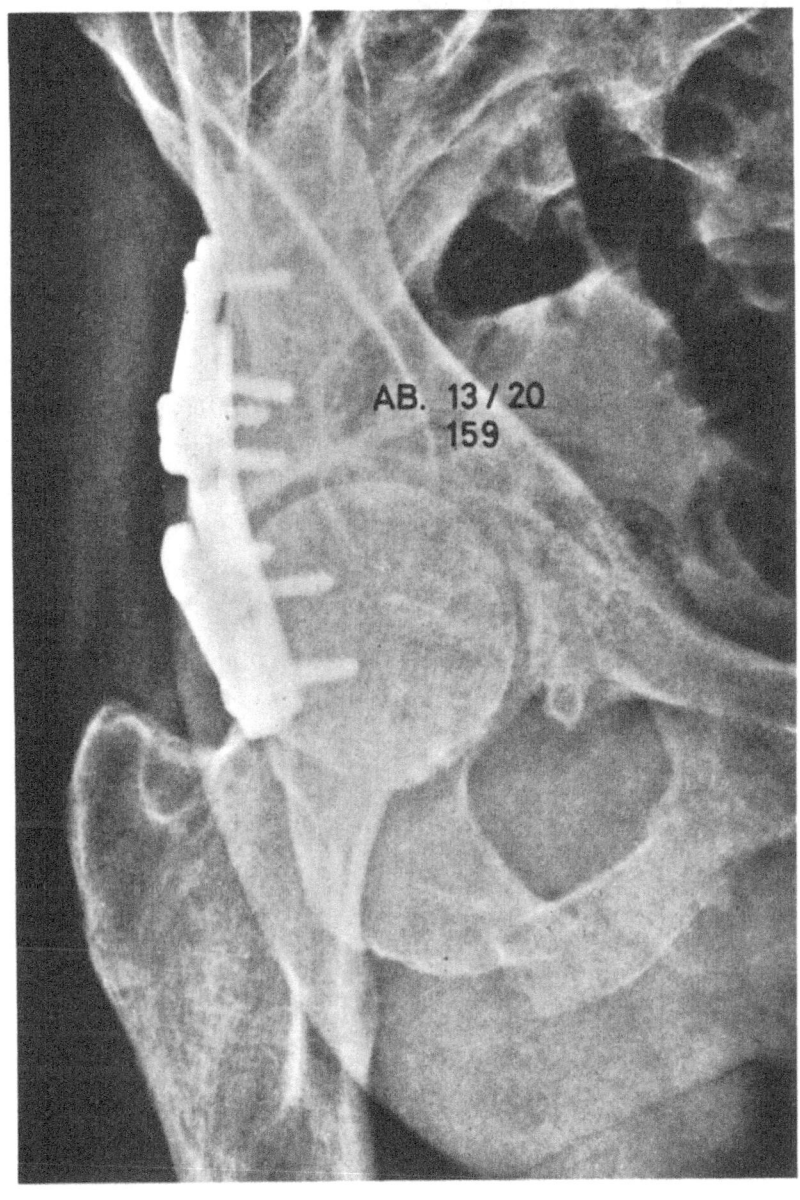

Fig. 26c   X-ray three years after the fracture. A full range of movement has been recovered in the hip joint

Concluding Remarks

The DCP was developed in 1965 and subsequently tested in 780 experimental fractures and osteotomies in a variety of animals: rats [30], rabbits [31], sheep [27], dogs and horses. Unrestricted postoperative weight bearing without external fixation devices was mandatory. The experiments performed with instrumented DCPs proved conclusively that compression and, therefore, stability of fixation were maintained. Clinical trials have been in progress since 1965 in one clinic and since 1969 in five clinics. First reports are very favourable. More than 1 500 human cases have now been treated with the DCP, and the plate has been released for general use.

References

1. MÜLLER, M.E., ALLGÖWER, M. WILLENEGGER, H.: Manual of internal fixation. Technique recommended by the AO-group. Berlin-Heidelberg-New York: Springer 1970.
2. BLOCK, W.: Die normale und gestörte Knochenbruchheilung. Stuttgart: Enke 1940.
3. PRITCHARD, J.J.: Histology of fracture repair. In: CLARK, J.M.P. (Ed.): Modern Trends in Orthopaedics, Vol. 4, pp. 69–90. London-Washington: Butterworth 1964.
4. COUTELIER, L.: Recherches sur la guérison des fractures. Bruxelles: Arscia SA-Edition 1969.
5. PERREN, S. M., GANZ, R., RUETER, A.: Mechanical induction of bone resorption. IVth International Osteological Symposium, Prague, Sept. 1972.
6. PERREN, S.M., HUGGLER, A., RUSSENBERGER, M., STRAUMANN, F., MÜLLER, M.E., ALLGÖWER, M.: A method of measuring the change in compression applied to living cortical bone. Acta orthop. scand. Suppl. **125,** 5 (1969).
7. PERREN, S.M., HUGGLER, A., RUSSENBERGER, M., ALLGÖWER, M., MATHYS, R., SCHENK, R., WILLENEGGER, H., MÜLLER, M.E.: The reaction of cortical bone to compression. Acta orthop. scand. Suppl. **125,** 17 (1969).
8. RHINELANDER, F.W.: Circulation of bone. In BOURNE, G.H. (Ed.): The Biochemistry and Physiology of Bone, Vol. II, pp. 2–76. New York-London: Academic Press 1972.
9. GANZ, R., BRENNWALD, J.: Recovery of medullary circulation of the osteotomy and internal fixation in the rabbit tibia. 31e Congrès de la Société Suisse d'Orthopédie, Réunion Franco-Suisse, Berne, mai 1971.
10. SCHENK, R., WILLENEGGER, H.: Zum histologischen Bild der sogenannten Primärheilung der Knochenkompakta nach experimentellen Osteotomien am Hund. Experientia Basel **19,** 593 (1963).
11. SCHENK, R., Willenegger, H.: Morphological findings in primary fracture healing. Symp. Biol. Hung. **7,** 75 (1967).
12. WILLENEGGER, H., PERREN, S.M., SCHENK, R.: Primäre und sekundäre Knochenbruchheilung. Chirurg **42,** 241 (1971).
13. ALLGÖWER, M.: Osteosynthese und primäre Knochenheilung. Langenbecks Arch. Chir. (Kongreßband) **308,** 423 (1964).
14. GALLINARO, P., RAHN, B., FILOGAMO, G.: The effect of compression in internal fixation of transverse osteotomies in rabbits (Abstract). Europ. Surg. Res. **1,** 171 (1969).
15. RAHN, B.A., GALLINARO, P., BALTENSPERGER, A., PERREN, S.M.: Primary bone healing. An experimental study in the rabbit. J. Bone Jt Surg. **53-A,** 783 (1971).
16. WIESER, C., ALLGÖWER, M.: Die Beurteilung der Knochenheilung nach stabiler Osteosynthese im Röntgenbild. Radiol. clin. Basel **31,** 297 (1962).
17. LANE, W..: The operative treatment of fractures. London: The Medical Publishing Co. 1914.
18. DANIS, R.: Théorie et pratique de l'ostéosynthèse. Paris: Masson 1949.
19. MÜLLER, M.E., ALLGÖWER, M., WILLENEGGER, H.: Technique of internal fixation of fractures. Berlin-Heidelberg-New York: Springer 1965.
20. EGGERS, G.W.N.: Internal contact splint. J. Bone Jt Surg. **30-A,** 40 (1948).
21. BAGBY, G.W., JANES, J.M.: The effect of compression on the rate of fracture healing using a special plate. Amer. J. Surg. **95,** 761 (1958).
22. TAMAI, T., HOSHIKO, W.: A new compression plate for osteosynthesis. Clin. Orthop. Surg. **2,** 941 (1967).
23. DENHAM, R.: Pers. comm.
24. LUHR, H.G.: Zur stabilen Osteosynthese bei Unterkieferfrakturen. Dtsch. zahnärztl. Z. **23,** 754 (1968).
25. MITTELMEIER, H.: Osteosynthese mit selbstspannenden Druckplatten. Bücherei des Orthopäden, in Druck.

26. BERTOLINI, I. A.: L'impiego della mia placca a compressione per l'osteosintesi dei vari tipi di osteotomie intertrochanteriche di femore. Clin. Orthop. **18**, 221 (1966).
27. PERREN, S. M., RUSSENBERGER, M., STEINEMANN, S., MÜLLER, M. E., ALLGÖWER, M.: A dynamic compression plate. Acta orthop. scand. Suppl. **125**, 29 (1969).
28. GALEAZZI, G.: Experimentelle Untersuchungen zur intraoperativen Druckveränderung bei der Plattenosteosynthese. Inauguraldissertation, Basel 1972.
29. VON ARX, CH.: Schubübertragung durch Reibung bei Plattenosteosynthesen. Inauguraldissertation, Basel 1973.
30. HUTZSCHENREUTER, P., Allgöwer, M., BOREL, J.F., PERREN, S.M.: Second-set reaction favouring incorporation of bone allografts. Experientia, **29**, 103 (1973).
31. RAHN, B., GALLINARO, P., HUNTER, W., SCHENK, R., PERREN, S.: Primary healing of osteotomies in rabbits using new compression plates (Abstract). Europ. Surg. Res. **3**, 170 (1969).
32. ALLGÖWER, M., EHRSAM, R., GANZ, R., MATTER, P., PERREN, S.M.: Clinical experience with a new compression plate "DCP". Acta orthop. scand. Suppl. **125**, 43 (1969).
33. ALLGÖWER, M., PERREN, S.M., MATTER, P.: A new plate for internal fixation – The dynamic compression plate (DCP). Injury **2**, 40 (1970).

Subject Index

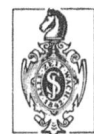

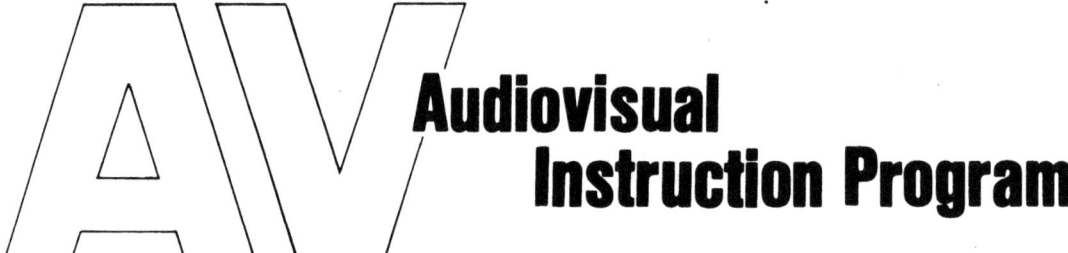

Audiovisual Instruction Program

Film Series: Internal Fixation of Fractures

**Internal Fixation
Basic Principles and Modern Means**
Medical advisors:
M. Allgöwer, Basle; S. M. Perren, Davos

Internal Fixation of Forearm Fractures
Medical advisors:
Th. Rüedi, Basle; M. Allgöwer, Basle;
A. v. Hochstetter, Basle

**Internal Fixation of Noninfected
Diaphyseal Pseudarthroses**
Medical advisors:
M. E. Müller, Bern; R. Ganz, Bern

Internal Fixation of Malleolar Fractures
Medical advisor:
B. G. Weber, St. Gall

Internal Fixation of Patella Fractures
Medical advisor:
B. G. Weber, St. Gall

Medullary Nailing
Medical advisors:
S. Weller, Tübingen; F. Schauwecker, Tübingen

**Internal Fixation of the Distal End
of the Humerus**
Medical advisors:
C. Burri, Ulm; A. Rüter, Ulm

Internal Fixation of Mandibular Fractures
Medical advisors:
B. Spiessl, Basle; J. Prein, Basle; B. A. Rahn, Davos

Forthcoming:
Corrective Osteotomy of the Distal Tibia
Medical advisors:
M. Allgöwer, Basle; Th. Rüedi, Basle

The Biomechanics of Internal Fixation
Medical advisors:
S. M. Perren, Davos; B. A. Rahn, Davos; J. Cordey,
Davos

Book and slides:

Manual of Internal Fixation
by M. E. Müller, Bern; M. Allgöwer, Basle;
H. Willenegger, Liestal

Films on Allo-Arthroplasty:
Total Hip Prostheses
(3 parts)
Medical advisors:
M. E. Müller, Bern; R. Ganz, Bern

Part 1: **Instruments. Operation on Model**

Part 2: **Operative Technique**

Part 3: **Complications. Special Cases**

**Elbow-Arthroplasty
with the New GSB-Prosthesis**
Medical advisors:
N. Gschwend, Zurich; H. Scheier, Zurich

Technical data:
Eastmancolor, magnetic sound, optical sound
16 mm, Super-8, EVR, VCR, TED-disc

All films available in English and German;
French versions in preparation

Sales:
Springer-Verlag, D - 1 Berlin 33, Heidelberger Platz 3

■ Please ask for special brochure

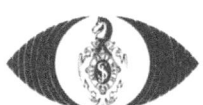

**Springer-Verlag
Berlin Heidelberg New York**
München · Johannesburg · London · New Delhi
Paris · Rio de Janeiro · Sydney · Tokyo · Wien